THE
BITTER
PILL

Also by Martin R. Lipp

RESPECTFUL TREATMENT
The Human Side of Medical Care

THE BITTER PILL

Doctors, Patients, and Failed Expectations

MARTIN R. LIPP, M.D.

HARPER & ROW, PUBLISHERS New York
Cambridge, Hagerstown, Philadelphia
San Francisco, London, Mexico City
São Paulo, Sydney

1817

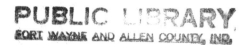
FIRST EDITION

Designer: Ruth Bornschlegel

Library of Congress Cataloging in Publication Data
Lipp, Martin R. 1940-
  The bitter pill.
  1. Physician and patient. 2. Psychotherapist and patient. 3. Physician and patient—United States. 4. Physicians—United States. 5. Psychiatrists—United States. I. Title.
R727.3.L55   610.69'6   80-7590
ISBN 0-06-012649-3

---

80 81 82 83 84 10 9 8 7 6 5 4 3 2 1

To my colleagues . . .
those who still take pleasure in conscientious
patient care, and those who continue to try even
when the process ceases to be pleasurable

and
to the memory of Mort, John, Phil, Ivan, both
Rons, Danny, both Steves, and the rest

Contents

Preface

This is a book about the doctor-patient relationship.

I have endeavored to go beyond the platitudes that state what the relationship should be, and write instead about what it has become—and is becoming.

In recent years I have talked with thousands of lay individuals and physicians about what is happening to this relationship. Though there are exceptions, the pattern seems clear to me. People are perplexed by what they see as doctors' callous behavior, and are furious at the medical profession generally. In turn, physicians feel themselves poorly understood by the public, often believe they are working themselves ragged without receiving appreciation for their efforts, and are increasingly resentful about what they perceive as a discrepancy between the demands and the rewards of their work.

I hope this book will provide a bridge between these polar views.

My intention is twofold: first, to give the thoughtful lay reader some understanding of what it is like to be a conscientious physician struggling to be a compassionate, technically competent, and socially responsible clinician. Why do there seem to be so few physicians like this? What happens to turn all the idealistic medical students into apparently brusque and insensitive doctors?

Second, I hope to offer physicians, medical students, and other health professionals greater understanding of their flagging morale from a broader perspective than is customary. Taking care of patients is enormously demanding work, made all the more difficult when persons bearing life-and-death-tinged responsibility are plagued with self-doubt and must labor in settings that promote mistrust.

I have approached these goals by telling a very personal story, building on my own experiences and those of other doctors I know, trying to piece together a pattern that places disparate elements in some sort of perspective. My primary focus is on psychiatry, in part because I am trained as a psychiatrist, and in part for reasons that will become clear in the chapters that follow.

My story is somber—an unavoidable consequence of the subject matter and the manner in which it has come to my awareness. The text begins with a physician's suicide, only one of many I could recount. During 1978 and 1979, I was chairman of the Well-Being Committee of our local psychiatric society, and in that capacity I accumulated a list of physician suicides. The doctors named in the dedication of this book are only a few among those whose suicides have had a personal impact on me. "Being a doctor may be hazardous to your health," read a cover headline in a recent issue of a widely read medical magazine. The crisis in morale is felt equally by physicians and by the public that comes to them for care.

This book has been in preparation for four years, and brewing within me for even longer. Many people—students, patients, friends, colleagues, family, and others—have contributed ideas, information, and support. I have tried to acknowledge printed resources in the Notes that appear at the back of this book. I have probably failed to recognize all the people who have been helpful, as the connection between contribution and source has blurred over time; but my gratitude goes to them all.

Various individuals have read the manuscript as it evolved and given freely and helpfully of their thoughts. I am especially grateful to Jerry Hannah and other members of the Asilomar Writers Consortium. I am also indebted to Suzanne Quick, Joan and Harrison Sadler, Stuart Schwartz, John Brosnahan, Jon Russ, Nina Mayer, Donna Buessing, Yvonne Knowles, Loma Flowers, Kenneth Woodrow, Steven Walsh, Phil Derbin, Paul Broeker, and Deborah Lipp.

Though I was employed by the Kaiser Permanente Medical Group and the University of California at San Francisco at various periods during the preparation of this book, it was written on my own time; and neither institution is in any way responsible for the content or opinions expressed in its pages. Nonetheless, my co-workers at the Kaiser Hospital in Hayward and my co-faculty in the Psychiatric Aspects of Medical Practice group at UCSF have continually stimulated my thinking and provided valuable collegial support, as have fellow members of the Well-Being Committee of the Northern California Psychiatric Society.

The research which was prefatory to the actual writing of the book was made significantly easier by librarians Alice Pipes, Jean Jones, Cindy Heathfield, and their respective staffs.

Two of my most valuable companions have been my typist, Margaret Oakley, and my editor, Ann Harris. Ann especially has helped me organize and develop my thoughts more fully than I would have otherwise. She has been my most critical reader, in the best sense of the word, and I owe her more than I can say.

Finally, out of respect for the privacy of people living and dead, both the individual psychiatrists, described by their first names only, and all the patients portrayed in the book, are freehand amalgams loosely drawn from aspects of people I have known. If you sought to put a real-life name on any one of them, you would seek in vain.

THE
BITTER
PILL

1 ALEX: The "Impaired Physician"

There was no doubt it was a suicide. There were empty bottles of Tuinal and Seconal at the bedside, which he had prescribed for himself on his own prescription blanks. The scrawled note at the bedside gave a cryptic message: "I've had enough."

Why did he do it? Alex was thirty-six. It seemed as if all the attractive rewards available to an ambitious, likable, and capable professional stretched inevitably across his future. He had an active and lucrative private practice, he gave his time generously at a low-fee community clinic, he taught at the nearby prestigious medical school, and he had recently published a well-received chapter in a well-received book. True, he had been divorced, from a woman for whom he still felt much love, but that was four years ago.

His friends regarded Alex as tough and smart and stable, someone who would not succumb to the kind of pressures that would bend ordinary individuals. His was a restless and moral intelligence: he constantly confronted his colleagues with the discrepancies between what needed to be done and what had not been done. No one had thought of him as weak or crazy or even peculiar. His death did and does stand out as a tragic loss. People of his caliber come along too seldom; we need all of them we can get.

When Alex's death became known, mutual pulse-taking among professionals in our community reached epidemic proportions. I received many phone calls, some from relative strangers, wanting assurance that I wasn't seriously depressed or suicidal. In response, I was righteously indignant: I was perfectly fine, I said. How could they even think such a thing?

The problem was, of course, that no one had perceived Alex as being suicidal. Several colleagues had even been with him a few hours before his death. Although they had chatted with him that very day, no one had guessed the imminence of suicide; no one had "diagnosed" his depression. Competent psychiatrists who make expert judgments about suicidal potential in their patients every day were totally unaware of the anguish and despair of someone they thought they knew well and cared about as a friend.

A secondary but by no means trivial problem was that a lot of people viewed Alex's suicide as a betrayal of a professional ideal. One of the psychiatrist's central tasks, after all, is to combat suicidal impulses and help sustain the life force when it is eroded by depression and hopelessness. If we can't buoy ourselves up when the going gets rough, how can we hope to help others? Alex's death was therefore not only a personal loss for his friends and a diagnostic failure for his colleagues, but it was also viewed by many as a slap at our profession. And psychiatry already has enough problems without being assaulted by the likes of Alex.

Ironically, the only people who had a premonition of the event were his patients: "Yes, he hadn't been his usual self for months. He had let himself go." Or, "The office was a mess. I had asked him if he were all right, but he smiled gently and said that my job was to look after myself."

The death was inevitable. If not Alex, then someone like him. Doctors, and especially psychiatrists, kill themselves all the time.

So what?

Why should you or any reader without a special interest in medicine or psychiatry care about the death of a single privileged and achieving professional? God knows there are enough other things competing for your attention and concern.

Alex is a starting point. More precisely, his suicide served as my starting point in a determined attempt to formulate and express the ideas in the pages that follow. Before he killed himself, I knew something was wrong, very wrong, with the way the physician's role is evolving in this country, but I couldn't put my finger on it. Now I think I can. At least I can come close.

The subject is untidy, involving so many people and so many conflicting facts and opinions and expectations that a full exposition of the issues would tax the most brilliant scholar—and I am not a scholar. I am a clinician. I spend my working days taking care of patients. I say this not as an apology but as a clarification. I think I have something important to say, and I have read it nowhere else.

As a clinician, I see patients mostly one at a time. My interest is in the individual and the particular, and that's how I think. Theories and statistics and research reports are of interest to me primarily as they help me to understand the singular circumstances of the singular individuals I see each day in clinical practice, and as they help me to understand myself.

That's how I've striven to write this book: using my individual experiences, and those of people I know, to try to make some general sense of fragments of experience. There are always loose ends, and everyone has his or her own perspective. The patterns emerge slowly, and sometimes not at all—but there are patterns, and in the repetitiveness of experience there is potential meaning and understanding.

Before Alex killed himself, I had known other physicians who committed suicide, and since his death I have learned of still more—a lot, in fact, by my standards. I will tell you about some of them as they become pertinent.

Alex's death was so upsetting partly because of the discrepancy between his public persona before he died and how he was viewed after death.

I had always thought of Alex as a special person. Damn it, he *was* a special person. I admired and respected him. I'm not a man who has heroes, and Alex wasn't my hero—but I looked up to him as someone with a little more guts than the average person, more idealism and more rigor in confronting the sorts of everyday struggles that give our lives meaning. I always felt that he was the kind of person I could depend on if I needed help from a friend.

When he killed himself, therefore, I was not only grieved, I was angry and resentful. He had his problems, of course, but so had I, and so does everyone else. How dare he abandon me like that? I had depended on him, and he had let me down. I still feel resentful to some degree. It's a selfish response, but fortunately not my only one. My thoughts and feelings are so complicated that it has taken me a long time to sort them out.

We held a psychological autopsy for Alex. A psychological autopsy, like a regular autopsy, refers to a process and an event. The process is a systematic investigation into the cause of death, as thorough and analytic as bright, concerned, and well-trained people can make it. Interviews with loved ones, colleagues, patients, and friends, anyone who seems relevant. An excavation of documents and files and papers. A search for clues. Why did this man do this thing at this time?

To the extent that a psychological autopsy refers to an event, it describes the congregating of all the people involved in the investigation and a verbal sharing of information and feelings, an opportunity for exchange and ventilation.

The autopsy for Alex involved a gathering of perhaps eighteen people. They were all decent and well intentioned, and I want to do them and their efforts justice; but inevitably, my anger interferes. In searching for explanations for Alex's suicide, these colleagues sought answers in the same way doctors usually do when they try to understand any death: they looked for evidence of disease. They dug deep within the man, searching for hints of dysfunction that would explain away his suicide and separate the man and the deed from the rest of us. They looked at quirks and traits that heretofore had seemed endearing and adaptive, and wondered if these could have been evidence of deep-seated pathology.

The search became a mission—and as is inevitable when investigators seek to confirm preconceptions, they found what they were looking for. Alex was sick, they said. Mentally ill. He had unresolved dependency needs. He was masochistic, self-destructive, and narcissistic. His suicide was a manifestation of temporary insanity. He had pathological idealism—whatever that is.

My colleagues and I were struggling to explain something beyond our grasp. They were no less stricken than I, no less anguished. We were doing the best we could with the tools of our trade, but I was profoundly dissatisfied with the results of the autopsy. My principal problem was that I had always flattered myself by thinking Alex and I were alike. If he was sick, then I too was sick—or so it would seem. Yet it has been my vanity never to doubt my own sanity. I think of my quirks and problems as normal quirks and problems, part of the human condition, not evidence of psychopathology.

The term *pathological idealism* grated. I had regarded Alex's idealism as one of his finest qualities, and I'm inordinately fond of my own idealism. We need all the idealism we can sustain, and in my obstinacy, I won't tolerate anyone evaluating Alex's idealism as pathological.

The observation that idealism was a factor in his death has a great deal of merit, but the ideals weren't unique to Alex. His ideals and expectations were a part of the culture we all shared, but for him they were more than platitudes. They were the standards that guided his behavior and doomed him to feel a failure.

He really believed that the doctor must always place the needs of the patient before his own. He really believed that the doctor must first do no harm. He really believed that the doctor-patient relationship was sacred, and that he had a responsibility to keep it so.

When he finally saw that he was doomed to fail, and that the failure would become more grievous with the inevitable flow of political and societal events, the meaning of his life eluded him, and he decided to end it. To compromise the ideals that were so important to him smacked of sacrilege, and a sacrilegious life was abhorrent. Throughout his youth he had wanted to be a superb, sensitive, technically competent, socially conscious physician and complete human being. He had been a doctor for ten years, and he finally understood that it was impossible.

You may have a difficult time accepting that it really is impossible for a doctor to be all those things. You may think that if doctors just tried hard enough—if their hearts were only in the right place, if they cared less about money—they could be anything that their patients wished.

Well, maybe some can, but most of us can't. Most of us are doomed to a failure of expectations. Alex's failed expectations led him to kill himself, and mine led me to write this book—a better and more productive choice, I hope. I am protected too by being a person who approaches compromise much more readily than did Alex, and I worry less about sacrilege. But compromises beyond a certain point take their toll in feelings of self-esteem, and you will learn about some of those as we go along. There are some things on which I won't compromise, but fewer than I once would have imagined.

Alex and I are not alone in our struggles. Over the past decade or so, there has been a growing rumble about a phenomenon that is generally identified as the "impaired physician" problem. It's something that was rarely discussed in public twenty years ago. Now almost every medical society, many medical centers, and some state licensing boards have set up committees to look into the problem and to serve as resources to "doctors in trouble." Some of this increased activity may be related to a greater openness about a phenomenon that has always been with us, but the greater openness is also a consequence of greater prevalence. The issue has become, if not respectable, at least unavoidable, because it is so widespread.

Increasing numbers of physicians feel overstressed and underrewarded, and foresee little prospect for constructive change within the practice of their profession. Like other human beings who feel trapped by the crosscurrents of external circumstances and personal expectations, more and more doctors have turned to traditional avenues of release: alcoholism, drug abuse, sexual adventurousness, and mental illness. A frightening number commit suicide.

In 1975 the American Medical Association held the first of what have come to be annual conferences on the disabled physician. The meeting was in response to a growing pressure, including an increasing volume of letters and phone calls from physicians and their families requesting the profession to *do something* about their plight.

People were stunned by what appeared to be the magnitude of the problem. Approximately 7 to 8 percent of all physicians are said to be alcoholics. Many have significant problems with drug abuse. The equivalent of one medical-school class each year is needed simply to replace physicians who commit suicide. How many more are there who don't come to official attention, or who are "impaired" in ways that are not so dramatic?

Throughout the conference, and in the publications that followed, the problem was discussed in terms of the "sick" or "mentally ill" physician. The medical profession could not see beyond its own frame of reference, beyond its own language and pathology-oriented approach, to view the problem in a broader context. Instead, as in the case of Alex, they focused on specific individuals, and applied diagnoses to them. They said these doctors were sick.

What you will read in the pages ahead is troubling. This is a book about the doctor-patient relationship, especially about what the doctor puts into it and gets out of it and how that is changing. It is a book about physicians who are struggling under the weight of criticism both from within and without—and the self-doubt and anguish they feel as they become increasingly aware that not only does much of the criticism have merit, but that the circumstances upon which the criticism is based are beyond the ability of any individual physician to change. My focus is on psychiatrists and, to a lesser degree, on others in the mental-health professions. Repeatedly, however, I will draw parallels between what is happening in psychiatry and what is happening in all other medical fields. Physicians in general are afflicted with high suicide rates and problems of alcoholism and drug addiction, and the phenomenon—by all accounts—is becoming more pervasive.

This is also a book about me. It started out as a book about issues, and I deliberately kept myself out of the text; but I soon discovered that I couldn't separate myself from what was happening to my colleagues, and I began to see my own life, and some of the career decisions I have made, in a different perspective.

This is a book about my friends and fellow professionals. After Alex's death I began to look more closely at other colleagues, to see if the stresses that had doomed Alex—and that I felt within myself—burdened others as well.

I would like to help you understand the quandary of the reasonably conscientious practitioners who care about patients as human beings, but whose performance nonetheless fails to live up not only to their patients' expectations, but also to their own personal expectations.

The major premise of this book is that there is a growing morale problem among those entrusted with our health care, especially physicians. Disillusionment and discouragement among doctors endanger all of us. Who will help us when we are sickest and most needy? What will sustain their dedication? What will fuel the emotional and physical energy the physician requires in order to care sensitively for the perilously ill, whenever and wherever needed, despite fatigue, frustration, and failure?

Those who think the question has a dollars-and-cents answer have fallen into the same trap as many in the profession. The problem is more subtle and complicated than that, and it is full of paradoxes.

Individually these paradoxes may not appear critical, perhaps no more than minor annoyances which any person with character should be able to shrug off. In sum, however, they are demoralizing for many in the profession.

Focusing on psychiatry is a useful way to begin, both because the paradoxes are more blatant and pressing in that field and because psychiatry—at its purest—embodies what many critics think is most lacking in modern, scientifically based American medicine: that intensely human relationship in which a sufferer communicates soul-deep, painfully private concerns to a healer who is the quintessence of patience, understanding, and caring.

2 CHRIS: Craftsman and Believer

Like Alex, Chris is a friend and a fellow psychiatrist, someone who cares deeply about patients and who works hard at being helpful. Until Alex's suicide, I never worried particularly about people like Chris. Now I'm not so sure. Sometimes I look at him and wonder whether he will be next. If not Chris, then who? It's a morbid preoccupation, searching for kernels of aberration in people you care about in order to predict potential suicide. Now I do it often.

Chris begins seeing patients at 7 A.M. five days a week and continues until 8 P.M. on Tuesdays and Wednesdays. He keeps these hours so he can see working people without disrupting their nine-to-five schedule.

He's on call twenty-four hours a day. He carries an electronic telephone pager on his belt, and he encourages his patients to call him whenever they need him. He may get called at any time: at a restaurant, in a movie, or during a quiet walk on the beach. He never has another psychiatrist take calls for him unless he is out of town. How could anyone else, who doesn't know his patients, give them the loving attention they deserve? He does not regard himself as a glutton for punishment; long hours and perpetual availability are simply expected parts of his work.

Chris's 7 A.M. patient three days a week is a woman architect who works in a prestigious San Francisco firm. Outwardly, she appears brusque, opinionated, intensely bright, in complete control of herself and her environment. Her co-workers regard her with a mixture of awe, respect, and fear; her temper and single-minded devotion to work are legendary within the architectural community. Her friends, the few that she has, see her as moody, often distant, easily hurt by criticism. Only she and Chris know that she keeps a loaded .38 revolver in her nightstand, not to repel possible intruders, but as the chosen instrument of her suicide. Three times a week as she leaves Chris's office, she says by prior mutual agreement: "I will not kill myself before our next appointment." According to Chris, she says that the only reason she is alive today is because of him; he has kept her from suicide on at least eight separate occasions. She has been seeing him regularly, sometimes as often as seven times a week, for five years.

How has Chris managed to save her life—if indeed her claim is true—and what do they talk about, these two, in all their hours together? Chris has no doubt. "I love her," he says, "and she knows it." What they talk about is the pursuit of personal meaning in the thousands of details of daily life. That's how he shows his love—by being a companion on an otherwise lonely quest for meaning in what is for her a disorienting contemporary culture. Chris talks about love with disarming simplicity. He loves all his patients, he says. He will see anyone who walks into his office for an evaluation, but he refers to other psychiatrists those individuals whom he feels unable to love. The ones he takes into therapy tend to fit a common cultural pattern. They are middle-class, highly educated, reflective, and interested in talking aloud about their inner struggles. Each is a rare jewel to him, multifaceted, whose exceptional worth becomes more evident the closer the scrutiny.

For years now, I have heard about Chris's woman architect and what he regards as her remarkable struggle to appreciate herself for the gem she is, and I don't know her name. I would never ask, and Chris would never tell me. Occasionally he will ask my advice about her in a collegial way—as I would and have asked his—and occasionally he will tell me about some particularly inspiring revelation that has grown out of their sessions together.

The word *sessions*—or the word *therapy*—seems a sterile way to describe what is surely a most intimate and evolving relationship.

Just two people in a room, one talking and the other listening, the latter every now and then making observations, asking questions, proffering a suggestion or interpretation. Chris helps people use their concerns to explore their souls, he says, on a journey to discover the nobility that he knows they will inevitably find. There are three levels of concerns. The first are the kinds of problems that are the stuff of everyday life: job hassles, people hassles, money hassles. He brushes these aside; they are mere details. Then there are the problems that one can discuss only with close friends if one is fortunate enough to have confidants: bitter personal disappointments, private sources of shame and guilt, paralyzing fears. These, he says, are only where he begins. The meat of his work concerns thoughts and feelings so deep within the individual that they may never have been expressed openly before, perhaps not even to the self. His job is to bring these matters to consciousness and help people come to terms with them.

Chris's office is in an old Victorian building whose whimsical yet genteel exterior suits his personal style. The building is in San Francisco's equivalent of Couch Canyon, a remarkable concentration of psychotherapists by any standard. The office itself is smallish, a bit on the dark side, with two comfortable, worn chairs on either side of a corner table, a writing desk against another wall, and even a working fireplace. The room is made intimate by dim lighting but is saved from seeming seductive by the piles of journals and books that line the shelves, cover the desk and table, and are stacked randomly on the carpet near the walls. Many are books on values and ethics, and others concern religion, philosophy, language, psychotherapy, anthropology, and history. Books on hard science and nonpsychiatric medical practice are conspicuously absent.

When Chris talks about loving his woman architect or his other patients, he refers to what others would call Christian love, or the love of a parish priest for his flock. Chris acknowledges the similarity but doesn't fret about it. He believes that the particular posture a healer maintains must suit his time and place, but is otherwise irrelevant. Healing abilities will find expression no matter what, and the labels one uses to describe the healers or their methods are no more than social conventions. He balks at using labels himself, but accepts that others may need them. When he sees a patient whose visits are paid for by insurance, he tells the patient that he needs to put a diagnosis on the insurance form. "Medical condition: anguished searcher.

Treatment: loving concern and patience," he would say if he felt free
to do so. Instead, under "Treatment" he writes, "individual psychotherapy," and he allows the patient to choose his or her own diagnosis.

Chris strives to maintain the most moral life he can; does he feel
duplicitous using diagnoses in such a slipshod and apparently dishon-
est fashion? He shrugs in response. "Diagnoses were created by people who need to chop things up in order to understand them. They
are all based on a limited view of humanity and a failure to appreciate the complexity of the interdependent factors that affect our
health. To diagnose my architect patient as 'depressed' implies that
her depression is a condition that can be separated from the rest of
her life, personal and family history, or the times in which she lives.
She is depressed because she is alive and sensitive to what is happening around her. Her depression is at once a symptom of her questing
and a stimulus to it. It's a tool she can use as she delves into herself.
But to call her depressed neglects all her other wonderful aspects, of
which she has so many that it would take me hours to tell you of
them. Her diagnosis is such an absurd simplification that I can't trouble myself to worry about it."

As Chris talks, leaning forward, furrowing his brow, gesticulating,
it's easy to get a sense of the charismatic optimism he must bring to
his patients. He says "questing" in three syllables: *coo-west-ing,* with
the emphasis on the middle syllable, conjuring up images of wagon
trains heading for the frontier in an epic journey.

"Don't you ever get discouraged, Chris?" I ask. "All those people
telling you their problems, hour after hour, day in and day out, week
after week?" He currently sees twenty-six patients, most of whom
come once or twice a week, and some three, four, or five times. Mostly
they come to talk about troubles, not successes. Nobody stops in to
say how good life is, how the kids are all getting *A's* or being voted
class president. Hour after hour, he hears about neglect, abuse, sad-
ness, hopelessness and helplessness. Many of his patients unleash
their anger at him, yelling and crying and demanding.

"Sure I experience turmoil with my patients," he says, "but I think
that's the only way to become a really good psychotherapist—by experiencing with my patients again and again the anguish of suffering
and the tumult of growth through suffering, as we both change. I
don't feel that I *am* a psychotherapist; I feel that I am constantly be-

coming one. That's what gives my work whatever specialness it has."

The process of psychotherapy is slow, frequently tedious, and rarely dramatic. Successes are often subtle. To attempt to capture the process here would make it seem simplistic or magical or fake.

Chris somehow manages to remain unperturbed, smiling, and optimistic. When I was practicing psychotherapy, I grew depressed if I saw too many unhappy patients. If my work and my personal life were in good shape, I could see perhaps ten people a week in psychotherapy without feeling burdened by the contagiousness of their troubles. I spent the rest of my professional time in briefer visits with more patients and in consultations that required limited involvement with patients. When things were not going well personally, I could barely tolerate seeing patients in psychotherapy at all. I didn't have enough reserves to sustain my patients and also give what was needed to friends, family, and myself.

"How do you do it?" I ask Chris.

He pauses, hunches up his shoulders, tucks in his chin, narrows his eyes. The effect is one of mock ominousness. He clamps onto my left forearm with his right hand, and growls: "I'm crazy, do you hear, stark raving nuts!" We laugh. This is not the first time we've had this kind of exchange. The irony for me is that he seems to believe his own assertion. He is one of the sanest, kindest and most decent people I know, with not a trace of malice in him, yet he frequently alludes to a dark core of insanity. When he says such things, I feel a stiletto of fear in my chest. Please God, don't let Chris become insane. I've seen too many healers fall apart, and too many kill themselves.

"You don't know what I'm really like, Marts," he says. Nor will he tell me. That's why he goes to his own therapist five times a week. Only his therapist knows about that side of Chris. Chris's visits to his therapist are not simply therapeutic in the conventional sense; they are also a continuing reaffirmation of his faith in the process. He views his own trips to a therapist, in part, as a public demonstration of confidence in his own profession. What is good for his patients is good for him, and vice versa. He attends his sessions religiously, and indeed to see him after a particularly productive session is to see an acolyte cleansed and serene. He believes profoundly in what he does and is deeply concerned for colleagues and friends like myself who suffer doubts.

He has been buoyed up by many successes, too. His architect patient is not the only person who thinks he is wonderful, a marvelous healing presence. He feels he has helped the majority of the people who have come to see him, and each success helps to sustain his confidence in his method of treatment.

Where he has not been helpful, he attributes the failure to extrinsic factors: a failure in his application of the method perhaps, an inability to continue using the method as long as the condition required, a failure of motivation on the patient's part, a lack of sufficient money to finance the amount of treatment required. But his faith in his method of treatment remains secure.

I've never seen Chris burdened by his work. He sees himself as an incurable romantic, a knight errant, jousting against the forces of evil within his patients, heroically rescuing them from their own dragons. He revels in his own heroism when he can and waits patiently when he cannot. He brings the same romanticism to his life. He approaches social occasions like an upbeat Fred Astaire—charming, witty, wearing white tie and tails on the flimsiest excuse, always ready for a spirited tango.

Chris is an exceptional person and an exceptional therapist. He has also been lucky: lucky in the stability of his beliefs and lucky in his ability to structure his practice to suit his interests. He sees whom he wishes, works in an office of his own design, and manages to avoid most external demands that would interfere with his relationship with his patients.

I both envy and resent him for it. By limiting his practice as he does, he focuses his energy on people most likely to respond positively to his ministrations. He gives enormously of himself in time and caring love, and in turn is rewarded by his patients with money and loving respect. It's a part of the bargain between them. He is lucky, and his patients are lucky.

3 THE DOCTOR-PATIENT RELATIONSHIP: Respectful Treatment

Chris embodies many of the expectations and aspirations I held when I entered medical school, yet which I have found increasingly difficult to sustain in our society. He loves his patients, and they presumably love him in return. I had thought that was what being a doctor would be like for me as well, but it's not. I'm fortunate that I like many of my patients, though the affection for the most part is superficial and limited deliberately to the professional setting.

Chris cloisters himself in a lonely office, seeing a few patients from a narrow socioeconomic stratum, charging them a lot of money, continuing treatment for years and years. He is an adherent of the psychoanalytic method, an approach to patient care that for me long ago withered from conceptual arthritis and lack of efficient applicability across a broad spectrum of patients—yet for him the approach seems to work. It's as though the 1960s and 1970s never happened to Chris. He doesn't worry about not seeing minorities or poor people, or the fact that he sees so few when so many others are suffering, or that the validity of psychoanalysis seems so much more fragile than it once did.

Chris is happy and apparently effective in what he does, yet there is something in his satisfaction and self-acceptance that I find profoundly upsetting. But I can't scapegoat him with it. It's not Chris. It's me. I would love to have the kind of intimacy with my patients that he does with his—at least, I think I would—but in order to do so I would have to renounce some allegiances that for me are equally compelling. I was raised with, and have consciously embraced, a set of values and social compulsions that essentially place Chris's style out of bounds for me.

I would feel guilty caring for the well-to-do when so many of the poor need access to a physician's skills. I have never felt comfortable turning away patients who couldn't afford my services, or letting my diagnostic or therapeutic efforts be limited by the patient's ability to pay. I have been a salaried physician since leaving medical school, and I expect to continue in the same pattern for the rest of my professional life. If there are economic impediments between the patient and ideal health care, the patient struggles with the institution that employs me rather than with me directly. This is an imperfect compromise on my part, but it remains one I can live with.

I also lack the emotional reserves to give my patients the accessibility and concern that Chris offers his. I can be caring and giving to patients for long periods of time, but those stretches must be finite, with clearly defined beginnings and ends. I find being on call twenty-four hours a day unendurable. The patients need so much that I have nothing left for myself or for my friends and family. Being on call twenty-four hours a day may make me a more complete physician, but it makes me feel less of a complete human being, a more limited family man and friend. I have chosen a path very different from Chris's, and from my moralistic perspective, a more virtuous one; yet I am not nearly as satisfied in my work as he is.

For the past dozen years or so, I have been very much preoccupied with the doctor-patient relationship: what it has been, what it is now, and how it is changing. I teach the subject to medical students, and I tour the lecture circuit talking about it to various medical groups. I have written a practical handbook for physicians on the doctor-patient relationship, *Respectful Treatment: The Human Side of Medical Care,* which embodies many of my experiences, biases, and recommendations. Lay people are usually fascinated by the title of my book. "Doctors certainly need to learn more about *that,*" they say. They regard me as though I am privy to information that is special and important and uncommon among physicians. I am simultaneously flattered and made uneasy by their praise. I know how little I know, and I know how often I feel inadequate. My credentials imply an expertise that is misleading, and my performance with patients seldom matches the standard that my reputed expertise would suggest.

The term *doctor-patient relationship* is subject to many very different definitions and interpretations. For me it implies an intimate bond between two people, built upon trust and mutual respect and shared experiences, enduring over time, and sheltered from external assaults by a sacred tradition which dates back over centuries and which spans diverse cultures.

Chris has that kind of relationship with most of his patients, and those relationships provide him with emotional resources to weather the inevitable ups and downs of a professional life—though he has not been subjected to the ultimate crisis of a patient's suicide. He finds strength in the solidity of his relationships with his patients, and the tradition of which these relationships are a part—and which he accepts unquestioningly.

My relationships with patients are different, substantially so, and so are those of most of my physician friends. We have lost much of our effectiveness as a consequence, and are more vulnerable in ways that we only dimly perceive.

I wouldn't be talking about the doctor-patient relationship, nor would you be reading about it, if it weren't for the fact that there is something in it that is important. Relationships matter, and the nature of a particular doctor-patient relationship can matter immensely when health—however broadly or narrowly defined—is precarious and the diagnosis uncertain or the treatment only marginally effective.

Part of the function of that special relationship is to help provide an atmosphere in which the patient will feel comfortable in self-revelation, where the patient will disclose the seemingly trivial bits of data that are relevant to an understanding of health and disease, where doctor and patient together can integrate information to form conclusions and to develop helpful strategies for diagnosis and treatment. Sir William Osler said, "It is much more important to know what sort of patient has a disease, than what sort of disease a patient has." The relationship is the key to learning about the patient, but it may also be the key to deciphering information relevant to the disease. So often the patient *knows* what is wrong with him or her in a way that the doctor does not. Deep down where the undiagnosable cancer grows, the patient knows what is wrong.

The relationship is simultaneously a source of potency in therapeutics. The potential for healing correlates not only with the patient's faith in the effectiveness of therapy, but also with the physician's faith in it and his or her ability to communicate that faith within a relationship which matters to them both. So much that is therapeutic occurs in the companionable silence that is shared by people who know and accept each other as valuable human beings, where there is time and a shared history which promotes reflection and a thoughtful exploration of alternatives.

That kind of relationship between doctor and patient is changing. Doctors are changing, and patients are changing. So, too, is our whole culture. Patients may feel they get less from their doctors than they got in the past, but doctors get less from their patients in turn.

That's what I resent about Chris. He has been able to protect himself from the changes and stresses that grind me down and that ultimately killed Alex, because he has in essence removed himself from what euphemistically is called our health-care system: that ponderous, maddeningly complex and confusing series of hospitals, clinics, and institutions where so much health care is given and received; those conflicting and demoralizing sets of expectations and rules and allegiances; those diffuse hierarchies and competing professions; those bewildering politics and administrative guidelines. Chris doesn't pay any attention to any of that. He works as a craftsman in an isolated workshop.

The irony is that he is a good doctor, some would say a very good doctor, and many would contend that it is a shame and a waste for Chris to confine his talents to so few patients. The paradox, however, is that if he tried to treat more people with a greater diversity of problems, people with whom he meshed less comfortably and over whose treatment he could exert less control, he would lose exactly those qualities that make him so admirable in his narrower context. What Chris can do for the carefully chosen few—provide highly personal, specialized care available twenty-four hours a day, day in and day out—he could not do for the many; and if he tried to provide highly personal, technically competent, accessible, comprehensive

care for the many, he might just end up killing himself. Perhaps literally.

No reader can take statements like this solely on the basis of faith,
or believe them simply because I believe them. More information is
necessary, so I want to tell you about David.

4 DAVID: The Cost of Caring

If you were to walk into David's office, you would sense immediately that the man's style is different from Chris's. David's office is located in a suburban building which houses other physicians and psychiatrists as well as a broad spectrum of business people and other professionals. The office itself includes a small waiting room; a large, bright consulting room with a separate exit so that persons leaving won't have to go through the waiting room; and a huge terrace, which is reached through sliding glass doors off the consulting room. The terrace has been imaginatively landscaped with abundant plants and a small fountain. To view it is to feel more tranquil. It's hard not to like the man who conceived of it and keeps it in such fine order. The consulting room itself contains David's chair set at an oblique angle to a couch, a handsome piece of living-room furniture big enough to accommodate several seated people. A large modern desk is off to one side with papers and desk paraphernalia neatly organized.

David is warm, affable, and easygoing. He laughs and jokes comfortably, with a keen sense of irony, a way of turning a situation inside out so that a burdensome problem seems less so. He is not nearly so private as Chris, and he and I have seen patients and families jointly. I know how he works, and admire his style. He nudges and ca-joles. He brings up information the patient has long since forgotten, and uses it to bolster a shaky ego or to suggest alternative responses to exasperating problems. He struggles alongside his patients with their difficulties of everyday living, helping them to view current stresses from multiple perspectives. He is far more pragmatic and less philosophical than Chris. He tries to help everyone who comes into his office, and will see any patient with any psychiatric problem. He prides himself on having a broad range of therapeutic skills, and ad-justs his treatment to the patient and the patient's complaints. He uses hypnotism when he thinks it will work. He uses behavior therapy when he thinks that appropriate. He prescribes medications when he thinks they are indicated, and he uses his own brand of Chris's long-term, insight-oriented therapy when that seems best.

David is a born helper. He really wants to help, and will go to extra-ordinary lengths to do so. With fourteen years of practice under his belt since medical-school graduation, ten since he finished his psychi-atry residency training, he has few illusions about curing people but believes fervently that most people can be helped. He doesn't like the term *healer;* it's too mystical for his taste. For David, treating people is the equivalent of helping them, and he believes that the term *ther-apy* is consistent in tone with the broad stream of helpfulness em-bodied by modern American medicine, of which psychiatry is a part. He sees himself as a doctor first and a psychiatrist second.

David regards himself as an eclectic psychiatrist—that is, one who has no firm roots in any single psychiatric tradition. He is not a Freudian or a Jungian, though he can talk knowledgeably about the writings of both schools and believes he has incorporated their most valuable ideas into his own clinical work. He has had only one crite-rion in the development of his techinques: will this help my patients?

David has one great weakness, and he knows exactly what it is. He wants so badly to help that he is vulnerable to feeling unworthy when he is unable to do this. The worst single week in David's life occurred when two of his patients committed suicide in separate and dramatic circumstances. It was tragic for the patients and ghastly for others concerned—but it was agonizing for David too. Soul-destroying.

The week began innocently enough. David had his usual Monday lineup of hourly sessions. He was scheduled to see six individual pa-tients and two couples, the latter for marital counseling, and he had an hour-long luncheon meeting at the local hospital, where he sat on the peer review committee. However, this Monday he was also "holding the butterfly net" for the local hospital, which meant that he would be responsible for walk-in patients who appeared to require hospitalization.

On this particular day, he was notified at 4 P.M. that such a patient was in the emergency room. "No rush," he was told. "She can wait until it's convenient for you to come over."

So at 6 P.M., after his last patient, he went to see what awaited him. The walk-ins were always interesting and frequently a challenge.

The patient was a young girl, not particularly pretty, rather pale and wispy, wearing a tattered flowered smock over faded and patched blue jeans, with an animal tooth on a chain around her neck. Her feet were bare and very dirty. She sat on a chair against one wall of the emergency room, swaying gently to a melody only she could hear. It was her smile that arrested his attention: a gentle, beatific smile spreading from extraordinary blue-gray eyes, and framed by a dramatic display of red hair.

She had been brought in by the police, who had found her wandering along the edge of the freeway. The officer who accompanied her had been concerned that she would wander into traffic. He had questioned her at length but without success. She had simply looked at him with wide eyes, flashing her incredible smile and occasionally swaying rhythmically to a barely audible hummed tune. She was pleasant and cooperative, but who or what she was eluded his understanding.

David fared no better. He sat with her for almost an hour, sometimes quietly, sometimes gently asking her questions, sometimes just sitting patiently, for a while even holding one of her hands in his own in an effort to establish contact. It was all in vain. She would do whatever he asked her to do—stand, turn this way or that, give him her hand—but she wouldn't speak or in any way respond to his questions.

What the hell should he do? There was no telling whether she had been like this for a few days or for a few years. She looked reasonably well fed and—except for the dirty feet—reasonably well cared for. Though her behavior was bizarre, he could not say with certainty that she was crazy—or psychotic, to use the technical term. However he proceeded, he would be operating on the basis of ignorance, intuition, and his concern for an apparently vulnerable stranger.

She looked so frail. If she left the hospital now, her future would depend entirely on the character and motives of the next person to take an interest in her. If someone kind, she would be all right for a while; if someone malicious ... he shuddered involuntarily. She would go uncomplainingly, wherever she was taken.

To hell with it, he thought. "Keep the patient's welfare primary," he mumbled, repeating the centuries-old mandate to physicians. He took out a 5150 form, an involuntary detention form, filled in the spaces, and signed it. Under California law, the young girl could now be held on a locked psychiatric ward for up to seventy-two hours. Technically, David had overstepped his authority. The relevant statute allows people to be deprived of their liberty on psychiatric grounds only on the basis of imminent suicide, imminent homicide, or grave disability, meaning inability to provide self with food, clothing, or shelter. David did not really believe that this girl's condition conformed to the criteria, but he felt that he couldn't in good conscience let her go out the door. Sometimes you just have to wing it, to take responsibility for doing what you think is right even though you know it stretches the law.

So he admitted her to the hospital as a "Jane Doe"; ordered some antipsychotic medications, which he thought would loosen her tongue; and left for home. It had been a long day, and he was tired and looking forward to relaxing over some wine with dinner.

Over the next twenty-four hours, the medication did its work. The girl became willing to talk, but only about selected topics. She did not want any more medicine. It filled up her head like resin, she said. She wanted to be released from the hospital. David talked with her during his lunch hour on Tuesday. She still refused to reveal anything about who she was, where she came from, or what her history might be. "Let me go," she said, slurring the words just a bit. David hated being in the position of jailer and tried to make his interest clear: "Look, my only concern is your welfare. You're a transient, and I'm certainly not going to get paid for taking care of you. I'm not into any power trips. After you leave, I don't expect to see you again. My only concern is helping you. I really, really want to help you."

"I'll be okay," she responded. Her eyes stared as wide as ever, but the smile was much thinner now, with just a touch of muscular tension around the jaws and temples. Was she tougher than she looked? Was she streetwise in survival skills beyond his comprehension?

"All right," David said. "I'll stop your medication, and if you still seem okay tomorrow, I'll sign your discharge." Her smile warmed up again, and as David rose to leave, she resumed her rhythmic swaying.

When he saw her on Wednesday, she was much the same as she had been the day before. She was still taciturn, but the smile had returned to full radiance. When he asked, "Will you be okay?" she nodded affirmatively. As she walked out the hospital door, he went over his mental checklist again. There was no reason to assume that so peaceful a creature would hurt herself or others; she looked as though she might be able to get by, however marginally. In the long run, this little piece of Dresden china would probably get broken apart by a life devoid of stability and protection, but there was nothing he could do. As it was, he had probably held her illegally for two days.

Two days later, on Friday, everything fell apart. Fridays were always depression derbies for David. He scheduled his most depressed patients for Friday so that he would have the weekend to recover. Depression was contagious. Whenever he saw several depressed patients, he always became depressed himself. The more depressed he became, the less energy and optimism he could bring to his patients but the more he could empathize with their experience. He used this insight and empathy, which was substantial in any case, to create a therapeutic bond with his patients.

"How do you manage to function as well as you do?" he would ask them. He focused on their valor, their achievements, however minor, which were gained with the flimsiest of motivations. He tried to convey to them an appreciation for their own ability, and let his respect for them nurture the roots of their own self-respect. But it was exhausting to listen to the litany of ego-destroying anguish, the suffocating unhappiness.

During his eleven o'clock appointment, the phone rang. Usually, after one ring, his combination answering and secretarial service would pick up the call. This time the phone continued to ring. He apologized to his patient, who was talking about a particularly painful exchange with her mentally retarded son, and picked up the phone. Betty, at his answering service, spoke in urgent tones: "I'm sorry to bother you, Doctor, but it's an emergency. The hospital wants you to come right away. One of your patients poured gasoline all over himself and set himself on fire."

"Oh, my God. Did they say who?"

"I'm sorry, the nurse just shouted into the phone and told me to get you immediately and then hung up. I think it was a man, but I'm not sure. You want me to cancel your afternoon appointments?"

"What? Oh, yes." He hung up the phone and turned to his patient. "I have an emergency—I have to go." He had been seeing this same lady for three years and never before had he interrupted a session. She was immediately understanding, her eyes alarmed: "I hope it's not ..."

She and David had talked about suicide many times. She knew that only one kind of emergency takes a psychiatrist flying from his office: someone somewhere was dead or on the verge.

As David raced his car toward the hospital, his mind careened through his list of patients. Who could it be? So many of them had come close to suicide at one time or another, but none had talked about planning so flamboyant a death as self-immolation on hospital grounds. Lester Robertson had been plagued by suicidal thoughts for months, but he spoke about the Golden Gate Bridge. Mrs. Lewis and Sally Touhey had both seemed better recently, and they were pill takers anyhow, people with histories of overdoses. Virgil Peters was always on the edge of suicide, but he was supposed to be in Montana visiting his mother. Maybe the trip had been devastating for him. Maybe he had come back early. Maybe ...

But when David arrived at the hospital, it didn't take long to find out. Someone had witnessed the whole thing from across the street, had seen a wispy red-haired girl walk to the center of the lawn, methodically bathe her body in liquid from a gallon jug, then take out what apparently was a butane lighter and erupt into a ball of flames.

He was her doctor of record, and it was his job to pronounce her dead. There was no doubt. Every bit of her was charred except for her own teeth, and the single animal tooth on a chain around her neck. Her hair was burned, her clothes, everything. The body was still smoking, and the stench of burned flesh was overpowering. He retched on the lawn, not far from the body, and was dimly aware that others had done the same before he got there. Everything was a blur. Later he would recall people in hysterics, and images of frozen expressions would assume stark clarity in his memory.

He spent the next several hours talking with the coroner's deputies, the police, hospital staff, the hospital director, the hospital attorney, reporters. By five o'clock he was exhausted, emotionally and physically. Every time he closed his eyes he would see her incredible eyes, the beatific smile, and a blaze of red hair suddenly erupting into flames.

Finally they said he could go. He called his answering service to let them know he was leaving the hospital for home. They needed to know where he was. A doctor is nothing if not responsible. No matter how tired you are, you always carry out your responsibilities. Betty was still at work, and she said she had some more bad news. The highway patrol had tried to reach him in the late afternoon. When she had explained that he would be tied up with an emergency for several hours, they had left a message, and Betty dutifully had taken down the details. A man had been seen jumping off the Golden Gate Bridge at 2:17 P.M. The body had not been recovered yet, but in the parking lot at the south end of the bridge, an unlocked car registered to Lester Robertson was found to contain a wallet with identification, and two letters, one addressed to the wife of the apparent victim and one to David. The note to David said simply: "My time is up, Doc. There's nothing more for either of us to do."

Somehow David managed to drive home. He remained composed, his face expressionless. The "great stone face," psychiatrists call it, the practiced therapeutic mask that hides personal feelings no matter what the patient may be talking about or what the psychiatrist may be experiencing internally. As he drove, David thought about Lester Robertson and what a decent human being he had been: a father who felt he had not done enough for his children, a husband who felt inadequate for his forbearing wife, an accountant who felt unworthy of the professional responsibilities he had been given. Yet the shortcomings were all measured by his own internal standards. The only criticism he received from people who knew him concerned his exasperating lack of confidence, his sensitivity to slights, and his brooding depression. With regard to others, Lester was unselfish to the point of self-sacrifice. David had been Lester's therapist for eighteen months, seeing him several times a week, hospitalizing him twice. Over the months, Lester had bared his most anguished thoughts to David. Sometimes David had cried along with Lester, as he struggled with the pain of his existence. Together they would smile sadly, and David would signal the end of the hour by saying, "Time is up, Lester."

David had liked Lester very much; he cared for all his patients far more than he liked to admit to himself. He would never use the word *love*; it was too corny. But how he cared. His chest had never hurt him as it did now.

As he walked into his house, he wondered if things would have been different if Betty had not called Lester to cancel his appointment that afternoon. Would Lester have lasted another day or another year? Or would it have made no difference at all?

He entered the kitchen, and as his wife turned to greet him, she immediately knew something was wrong. "Hold me, honey. Hold me." His voice quavered and he started to sob—deep, gasping sobs. "Hold me, hold me." It was a long time before the tears stopped.

By Monday he was back in his office, seeing patients again. They needed him. He was sure of that, even as he was sure of his own need to be needed. But things were different. He had girded himself with a thin layer of emotional armor. He would never be quite so vulnerable to his patients again.

Sometimes David and I get together for coffee and shop talk, and to outward appearances he seems the same: easygoing, witty, comfortable with himself. But every now and then, when we're talking about one of his patients, tears come to his eyes in a way they never did before.

On these occasions I'll ask him: "Are you okay?" And he'll respond, "Yes, I'm okay."

"Then what are the tears about?"

He'll look at me with a smile, and say, "There's nothing wrong with tears. A little bit of crying wouldn't do you any harm either, you know."

I nod and ask, "If you ever contemplate suicide, would you please let me know? I'd really be furious with you if you knocked yourself off without clearing it with me first."

"I'm okay," he says. "Don't worry about me."

But I do.

5 THE DOCTOR-PATIENT RELATIONSHIP: Setting Emotional Limits

I worry about David and he worries about me. I think he becomes too involved with his patients, cares too much about them, puts himself inordinately at risk—and he thinks I am too fearful of becoming involved with patients, that I maintain too much emotional distance from them. He thinks that I have dropped out of psychiatry, and that concerns him as well.

I am a fully trained and board-certified psychiatrist, and I teach in that capacity at a medical school; but I don't practice the kind of psychotherapy that is the principal stock in trade of most psychiatrists. When I see patients, I do so as a general practitioner in what is a combination emergency room and drop-in clinic. I take care of patients with broken arms and heart attacks and stuffed noses as well as those with nervousness and depression and psychosis.

However, I use my psychiatric training on a daily basis. I listen to my patients more comfortably and acceptingly than do most nonpsychiatric physicians I know, without any compulsion to have answers for every problem. I trust my patients more, and I'm much more accepting of the self-centered and cantankerous behavior that illness often generates in people. I understand the usefulness of simply sitting with patients and their families through tears and anger and other forms of emotional release. And I understand, in a way that some doctors never learn, that my most important tool with patients is myself, my own feelings and perceptions and reactions, and I constantly strive to use myself as effectively as possible. When I see a woman with pneumonia, for example, I try to be sensitive to how this disorder in this person at this time will affect her personal and social life, even though often there may be little I can do about it. If the same person comes in after a suicide attempt, I sew up her slashed wrists as well as talk with her about the woes that led up to her desperate gesture.

The breadth of my professional work is therefore much greater than David's or Chris's. Chris sees perhaps thirty to fifty patients a year, David sees that many in a month, and I see about that many each day, averaging one patient every ten to fifteen minutes over a twelve-hour day.

I have chosen my particular professional path for a variety of reasons, some quite personal and some less personal and more related to what I perceive as political realities. I'll discuss some of those in the pages ahead. The point to be stressed here, however, is that different practice settings and differences in specialty focus have implications for each physician as a human being. Each setting has different emotional requirements and different potential rewards.

When I first entered medicine, I took the doctor-patient relationship as a given, much in the same way I might regard a clock or a calendar. My relationship with my patients was, like time itself, simply an unalterable element of my daily work. I assumed that doctors who were basically likable—as I perceived myself to be—would get along comfortably with patients and without any fuss or effort; and that those doctors who were not naturally likable were the people who would have difficulty relating to patients.

As I talk with lay people now, I find that many, perhaps even most, have the same general perception. Doctors who are easy to get along with are seen as being inherently "nice," and doctors who are not so easy to get on with tend to be classified in terms of derogatory labels: "insensitive," "uncaring," "arrogant."

There is relatively little appreciation for the fact that doctors who are perceived as "nice" usually have to work very hard to achieve that effect, or that doctors who are regarded as "not nice" by some patients may be considered "very nice" by an equal number of others. What is missing in the general view of the doctor-patient relationship is an appreciation for how variable an individual doctor's behavior can be, and the myraid factors that can and do affect it. Much of that variation depends on the patient's personality (or that aspect of it which is most apparent on a given day), as well as the complaint or circumstances that bring the patient to the doctor. Even more important are the vast number of expectations and pressures that, though external to a given doctor-patient relationship, nonetheless have enormous potential impact upon it.

Many of those factors will become more obvious in subsequent chapters. For now, I would like to stress two points. First, no doctor can care compassionately about all patients equally at all times. The emotional cost is too great. There are too few happy endings. Suffering and the potential for death perfuse the doctor's every working day.

I still remember the first patient of mine who died. I was in medical school at the University of Nebraska, a student on one of the wards at the Douglas County Hospital in Omaha. He was an old man, a weatherbeaten, cantankerous Nebraska alfalfa farmer dying from cancer of the pancreas. He had outlived all his relatives and friends, and no visitors came to see him. There was no cure for his disease, and, since I felt I had little else to give him, I spent whatever spare moments I had just chatting with him. Mostly I listened, as he talked with a trace of a Scandinavian accent about what it had been like to live through the last thirty years of the nineteenth century and the first sixty years of the twentieth. I was with him when he died, his hand clasping mine so hard that it seemed I could feel it for weeks afterward. I felt empty and helpless. Over the years since then, dozens of my patients have died. I don't know the number, and few of them stand out in my mind. There have been too many, and there will be many more.

Yesterday another one died. She was thirty-five years old, someone unknown to me before she became my patient. I still remember her name, though mercifully I know I will soon forget it. Forgetting is a professionally acquired skill, and I have worked at it.

The moment I saw her, I knew she was sick; but I didn't know she was going to die. She asked me, "Am I going to be all right?" And I said, "Yes, you are going to be fine. We're going to help you as best we can." And I did my best, in caring for her and in keeping her husband and two daughters informed about everything I was doing. If I had been able to diagnose more quickly the fulminant infection raging in her heart, perhaps she would have lived. If she had seen a doctor other than I, perhaps she would have been healed.

Might-have-beens make no difference. She came to me for help, and she is dead. I didn't kill her, but I didn't save her either. I saw forty-three patients yesterday. She was number thirty-one. I remember the names of none of the other patients I saw that day. It may be weeks or months before another of my patients dies, or it may be tomorrow. It's just a matter of time. That's part of what being a doctor is about.

I pronounced her dead at 9:11 P.M.; and after that I saw twelve more patients before going home at midnight. None of them knew I was brooding about my thirty-five-year-old lady, and what I might have done that I did not do, and what I had done that in retrospect I think I should not have done. My clinical productivity and personal happiness depend on not remembering the death too long; but I can't forget too quickly either. My humanity depends on that.

Paradoxically, if I am sensitive and caring with all my patients, I open myself up to more emotional wounds than I may be able to bear—yet if I close myself off to some or many of my patients, if I cease being sensitive and caring beyond a certain indefinable level, then I cease being the kind of doctor I want to be. I relinquish those personal qualities that give my professional life much of its meaning.

The issue of meaning brings me to another point I want to stress: the multiplicity of motives that lead doctors to take care of patients. Superficially, people become physicians for the same reasons that they embark on arduous courses in other ambitious endeavors: money, status, social contacts, a work identity in addition to a personal one, and a desire to achieve mastery over challenging problems that capture their imagination. Granted this, what qualities, what personal rewards do conscientious doctors seek in their contacts with patients as human beings, day after day after day? Where do they attain the sense of meaningfulness in their work? Chris sees himself as an artist in the use of a technique and wants to apply that artistry to transcend mundane obstacles so his patients can achieve insight and enlightenment. David, above all, wants to *be* helpful and to *feel* helpful, and he is flexible in how he achieves this. Some doctors get pleasure from possessing and applying arcane knowledge, or by being parental or pedagogical with patients, or technically adept with complicated equipment or procedures, or popular with large numbers of patients, or gaining the respect of their peers.

All this sounds so straightforward that we can easily mislead ourselves into thinking it is simple. The kinds of rewards a physician seeks will influence his or her behavior with patients, however subtly, producing incremental changes that result in greater or lesser satisfaction for the parties involved. The patient too comes with a set of expectations, seeking certain kinds of rewards in visiting the doctor. Some patients want tender healers, others wish stern authority figures or accepting parents or adept technicians, in varying mixes. Oftentimes, these wishes are only vaguely understood, and both doctor and patient are seldom able to articulate exactly what they seek at any given time. Moreover, each person's needs change as circumstances change.

One classic example concerns a patient who is mentally and physically able to take care of her own chronic arthritis but who comes to see a doctor for emotional support and reassurance, and because she would like to feel approval and affection from her doctor. If she is cared for by a skillful but standoffish physician who values objectivity and personal distance as a means of pursuing scholarly problem-solving, there is bound to be a clash between the two.

The opposite can easily happen too. I have seen many patients who become wary and evasive when I seek to get to know more about them than they feel is relevant to the complaint they have presented. For instance, a wiry, intense man of thirty-one came to see me, ostensibly for headaches. I inquired cursorily about his job and living situation and learned that he was a bus driver on a troubled route plagued by teenage vandals, and was simultaneously trying to start a new occupation as a real-estate broker. He was working fourteen hours a day, seven days a week. There was no doubt in my mind that stress was playing a role in his headaches, but the patient refused to discuss the matter: "Look, Doc, what I came here for was a prescription for some pain medicine. If you aren't going to give me any, why don't you just say so and let me be on my way."

There was nothing inherently wrong with my patient wanting a prescription for codeine, or in my wanting to have some impact on his personal life so his headaches would decrease; but we were both wasting our time and risking ill feelings until we could agree on some shared goals.

The diverse motives within and between doctor and patient are not in themselves either good or bad. What is important is the match between the participants, and a sensitivity in both parties to the variety of intrinsically sensible motives that can bring them together, yet nonetheless lead to strife.

As each physician begins to sense that his or her own values can be at odds with those of the patient in any given circumstance, the doctor must learn to seek compromise solutions. To develop compromises, however, usually requires effort from both parties, and a generosity of spirit.

The nature of those compromises therefore depends in part on the doctor's readiness to make concessions and to offer an extra measure of creativity and concern, and ultimately on the doctor's personal resources. Those who are emotionally secure usually have more emotional reserves to share with patients and can afford more generous compromises. Those who are under stress—or feel emotionally deprived—often have less to give.

Yet we are all under stress from time to time, and those sources from which all of us draw nurturance are under extraordinary stress too: the family as an institution, the doctor's spouse as a reliable source of support, the community and neighborhood as stable entities. Feelings about the importance of work and profession versus nonwork activities and our sense of what is worthy of respect in the eyes of fellow citizens can no longer be taken for granted. Today, each individual physician operates on a much less stable base of assumptions and support than in the past.

Physicians start learning about making compromises in medical school, and the process leaves few illusions.

6 SALLIE: Great Expectations

I first met Sallie when she was in her third year of medical school. She had heard me give a lecture, sat in on a few of my classes, and came to ask my advice. She had decided to go into psychiatry, she said. How frank should she be about her own experiences as a psychiatric patient, hospitalized against her will?

I saw before me a young woman in her early twenties: hair in braids framing her head like a halo, leather sandals, wraparound print skirt, and dark tank top. Over her own clothing, she wore the white coat of a medical student. Like many of her classmates, she carried her books in a bright blue nylon backpack slung over one shoulder. She seemed so young and so earnest.

We talked for a long time. Sallie portrayed herself as an intellectual, outspoken, physically awkward child, born to a family in which these qualities placed her at odds with everything her parents sought for her. They wanted her to find happiness in ways that they understood and through avenues they had worked hard to make accessible to her, a world of private academies, of country-club dances and chic hairdressers, and of studied and conspicuous leisure, of elegance and grace and charm.

Sallie's failure as a debutante was as painful to her as it was to her parents. Her body was flat where it should have had curves. Her skin had the tint of manila folders rather than rose petals; where others glided, she tripped and stumbled. Her parents ached for her and responded to her evident shame and guilt by giving her more advice and working more feverishly to mold her to their dreams.

In college Sallie made a tentative decision to stop trying to be something she could not be and instead take advantage of her obvious strengths in science and mathematics by going into engineering. She loved her parents, as they loved her, but it was a love tempered by a growing awareness of how their interests and values diverged. Her mother and father were appalled. Spending time in an overwhelmingly male engineering school would simply serve to exaggerate what they considered to be her insufficiently feminine qualities. They could not see how she could find happiness in such a path. They stopped short of forbidding her choice, but their disapproval was so patent that Sallie felt paralyzed. She grew listless and depressed, doubted her own worth and that of life itself, and took an overdose of her mother's sleeping pills.

She spent the next two months in a psychiatric hospital. Though the hospitalization resulted in a clarification of her own priorities and a strengthening of her resolve to pursue them, she believed that her progress came despite the treatment program rather than because of it. Her greatest teachers were her fellow patients. She hated her doctors' control over her, hated the medications that blurred her mind and made her more pliable, hated the tube feedings she endured when she refused to eat, hated the master-slave mentality that she felt pervaded the so-called therapeutic relationship. Most of all, she hated the fact that her parents had been able to commit her to a hospital against her will. Though the medical care had saved her life, she saw the extended hospitalization principally as punishment for a chain of events that were as much the responsibility of her parents as herself.

When Sallie got out of the hospital, she returned to school and embarked on premedical studies. Her parents were less than joyous, but felt this to be an improvement over engineering; and they were now much less certain of their own role in mapping out choices for her. As their confidence ebbed, hers flowed. Out of her own experiences she developed a steely determination to bring noncoercive healing to others, an abiding skepticism about the wisdom of people in authority, and a certainty that patients often know more about healing than do doctors.

Sallie's college performance was simply stunning. She was a straight-A student, an exceptional accomplishment at a respected and highly competitive school. In addition, she participated—often in a leadership role—in the proliferation of protest movements that were a part of campus life in those days when the Vietnam war was so anguishing.

Despite her history of psychiatric hospitalization, she had no difficulty getting into medical school. In addition to her grades in college, she had near-perfect scores on the Medical School Admissions Test; and while she had made enemies with her outspoken opinions, she had also won respectful and enthusiastic supporters among the faculty. The letters of recommendation to medical school all struck the same chord: this student has the potential to make an outstanding contribution. Her unique blend of brilliance, courage, and moral outrage will shake the system and improve it at the same time.

By the time I met her, in her junior year, she had developed a good but not exceptional academic record. All her classmates had been *A* students in undergraduate school too, and Sallie was finding the competition more rigorous than she had expected. Nonetheless, she was able to bring a special empathy to clinical work; few of her classmates could match her understanding of sickness and hospitalization as seen through the patients' eyes.

"That's one thing I can be confident of," she said. "I'm sensitive to the patient's experiences. That's something I don't need to be taught, I don't need to learn, because it's already a part of me and my experiences."

But Sallie changed during the first six months of her junior year in medical school, when she began to take actual responsibility for people who were ill. There were so many sick people to care for, and so many details to master with each. Every morning she and her intern and resident would make rounds of the ward, to see their charges. On an average day there were thirty such patients. If Sallie's team spent only five minutes with each—listening to heart and lungs, reading new entries in the chart, assessing laboratory tests—the process of making morning rounds took two and a half hours. There was no time for in-depth talk with any of the patients. Everywhere she turned, there were demands on precious minutes. Reading conscientiously about the voluminous details of a given illness and its care took time. Drawing blood took time. Doing a spinal tap took time. Going to look at X-rays took time. Often the processes were delayed by the inertia and complexity of the hospital itself, which seemed to conspire to make sure that equipment and people were never readily accessible.

At night she dreamed about the clutter of her professional life. The skies of her dreams were filled not with stars but with ions, electrically charged chemical particles whose concentration and whereabouts were important to her patients' care. Clusters of potassium, sodium, and bicarbonate would twinkle, and the dreaming Sallie would chase after first one and then another, with the one out of her grasp always seeming the most important.

She dreamed about cardiac arrests and operations and electronic equipment and medications and diseased organs, and of course she dreamed about the patients she saw during the day.

There was the heavy equipment operator with the recurrent chest pain. He was a huge man with granite features, beefy complexion, and leathery palms. Everything about him radiated fierce pride and independence. He resented the fact that his chest pain kept him from his work, hated being in the hospital, and distrusted his doctors. He believed that his previous experience with medical care had been unsatisfactory, and he expected no more of his stay at this hospital. He was angry and accusatory, and Sallie found him difficult to like. Nonetheless, she could understand that his illness threatened his independence, that he felt awkward and vulnerable in the hospital's unfamiliar milieu, and she didn't take his anger personally. She hoped that she could help make his hospital stay go smoothly.

He had come to the university hospital for evaluation preparatory to open-heart surgery. He expected to receive cardiac catheterization for diagnostic purposes and then meet with the surgeons to hear their recommendations. The whole process should have taken two or three days. But the preliminary X-rays and other tests which he had brought with him from his community hospital three hundred miles away seemed inadequate in a number of respects. They all had to be repeated, and that alone took three days. He was scheduled for catheterization on the fourth day, but the machine broke down and was not fully operational until too late on the fifth day to do Sallie's patient any good.

The catheterization team did not work on weekends except in the case of emergency, and he did not qualify. He was scheduled for catheterization on Monday, the eighth day, but two emergencies took precedence. On the ninth day the procedure finally took place, but the pressure readings were inconsistent, so the procedure had to be repeated the following day when a more experienced technician was available. At each stage the patient's rage mounted, and Sallie got the brunt of it. She could understand his feelings and understand the problems of the system, yet she was caught in the middle. There was nothing she could do but feel inept and powerless. Finally the procedure was completed satisfactorily, and the patient stormed out of the hospital. He couldn't stand being there any more. He would come back the following week for the conference with the surgeon.

But he didn't. He had a massive heart attack while mowing his lawn and died instantly.

Sallie discussed the evolution of events with me in painstaking detail. What could have been done differently? How often could she struggle with such events and still retain a reservoir of sensitivity for the next patient who came through the hospital's door?

Sallie began scaling down her expectations of herself. Her patients were all strangers when she met them; she began to accept that most would remain strangers all the while she was caring for them. How could it be otherwise? They came from diverse cultures and experiences; to understand them as people, one had to also understand the context in which they lived—and there clearly wasn't time or opportunity for that. It wasn't as though Sallie had grown up with these people, gone to their churches and picnics, known their families, heard about their forebears, seen them in their homes and at work. The stereotyped general practitioner of previous generations never needed to take a history. He had lived history with his patients, and their lives were intertwined. Sallie has no such advantage. If she were to attain any sort of comprehensive knowledge about her patients, she would need to accumulate that knowledge bit by bit, scrap by scrap. She would not only need lots of time with each patient but time too to chat with families and teachers and friends and employers and often police and social workers as well.

Instead she narrowed her scope to strictly medical aspects of patient care, though she continued to keep alert to patients who were particularly needy. If she couldn't have in-depth relationships with all her patients, she could have them occasionally—at least she could try.

"This time pressure is ridiculous," she said, looking at me gravely. "They make special efforts to select well-rounded people for medical school, and then the process of training and the demands of getting through it systematically force you to be narrow."

No matter how much she tried to identify with the patients, to remain partisan to them and their experience, she found herself often incorporating the thinking and values of her colleagues and mentors, the other students, interns, residents, faculty, and staff. All too frequently, she thought of patients as the great "them," a mass of needs and demands and complaints. When she worked at it, she could overcome this tendency; but she was surprised that she could no longer take her compassion and empathy for granted.

The most agonizing experiences for Sallie came when she began to accept the necessity of treating people against their wishes. Her first such challenge was a pediatrics patient.

Sallie was in the emergency room when an ambulance brought in a four-year-old girl who had been hit by a car while running away from a baby-sitter. Her forearm was bent at a crazy angle and she had bruises on her chest and abdomen. The youngster screamed in pain and fear. "I want my mother, I want my mother," she wailed. Sallie did her best to calm the child; so did the baby-sitter and the nurses and doctors—but the efforts were in vain. Despite their shared sense that it was better to proceed with the patient's understanding, their urgency overcame their scruples: she could bleed to death internally while they tried to reason with her. Sallie swallowed her loathing of involuntary treatment and helped hold the child down while the intravenous was started, blood tests drawn, pain medication given, and the patient prepared for surgery. What else was she to do?

Later a man in his thirties was brought in, gaunt, jaundiced, and frail. He had metastatic cancer, which had spread to his liver and brain. He was confused and disoriented. He paced restlessly, randomly, and because his coordination was faulty, he kept falling. The man's family knew he was dying and wanted to keep him at home, but they were emotionally and physically at the end of their resources. They couldn't watch him twenty-four hours a day, and God knows what would happen to him if they let him out of their sight for a moment. His energy seemed inexhaustible for such a fragile skeleton of a man. He was doing such bizarre things: he put a woven reed basket on one of the stove burners and lit the flame. There was a little baby in the house, and the man seemed strangely intrigued by its face and kept jabbing at it with his index finger. The wife was terrified that he would hurt the child, poke out its eyes. Couldn't the doctors give him something to make him sleep at least a little while? He refused to take any medications. Despite his protestations, Sallie and the intern ordered sedation and helped hold the struggling patient while the nurse gave the injection. What else was there to do?

Sallie felt herself becoming what she had always thought she wanted to become: a professional—but in the process, she began to see her role in a new and unexpected way. She had to accept the reality that her training would help her see disease and its treatment in a way that might conflict with her patients' views.

Her understanding was at once deeper and narrower than theirs. She comprehended so much more, she had mastered such great detail, and it was bound together in so intricate a way that she often felt at a loss to explain a given disease to the patient in whom it resided. She understood that a disease and its treatment were only one aspect of a patient's life, and that it was the patient—not the doctor—who would usually have to make decisions about how realistically a given treatment fit into his or her life. The doctor could only recommend.

Yet sometimes Sallie did more. Sometimes she intruded her expertise into patients' lives. She started intravenous treatment on patients who were terrified of needles, and did so over their protestations because she knew it could be life-saving. She did painful bone-marrow aspirations on people who had no tolerance for the procedure, for the same reason. She sewed up lacerations on thrashing drunks in the emergency room, and did spinal taps on uncooperative people with head injuries, all with grim determination and with a growing conviction that sometimes the doctor knows best. In the instance of conflict between doctor and patient, the doctor's professional expertise must often prevail for the patient's own good.

Sallie did not like what was happening to her. She felt herself changing in ways that she only dimly understood but was beginning to perceive as a natural consequence of caring for perilously ill patients. She sensed that she was erecting an emotional barrier between herself and her patients; she was afraid to do otherwise, but she didn't like it.

Laboring under the weight of the changes that encumbered her, she looked around for heroes and heroines ahead of her in their training. Where before she had wondered why the empathetic and optimistic students turned into such cold-fish interns and residents, she was now beginning to understand.

In coming up against her limitations so abruptly—and in doing it at such an early stage in her career—Sallie felt a pervasive sense of failure. Even though she had planned from the first to specialize in psychiatry, she had assumed that being a humanistic, patient, and technically competent generalist was something she could do with ease. She was aghast at how difficult all that seemed to be.

In nonpsychiatric work, she made the decision that was so distressingly common among her classmates: when you haven't got the emotional energy and time to be both technically competent and humanely compassionate, sacrifice compassion to competence. She measured her progress through medical school the same way most students do: by how many IV's she had started and how quickly she could start one under pressure; by how much she knew about intracellular metabolism and beta-lipoproteins and obscure drugs—and how articulately she could present her knowledge to her professors; and by how much "pathology" she had seen and could recognize, entirely separate from the identity of the patients in whom the diseases resided.

She remembers how pragmatically she had responded to advice when she failed to identify a cancer of the prostate in a male patient who was her responsibility. The surgical resident who supervised her had discovered the problem during his own examination of the patient. He told her that next time there might not be someone to do an exam after her, that next time the responsibility would be all hers, and that she couldn't afford to be inexpert in doing rectal exams.

"There are thirty-two men on this ward," he told her, "and each one of them has an asshole. I want you to stick your index finger up each one until you know how to tell the difference between a normal and a diseased prostate."

She did as she was told, even though she felt that both she and the thirty-two men were somehow dehumanized in the process. She did it because she thought it was necessary to her own medical-school survival, and for the benefit of future patients. Even when she became a psychiatrist, she could expect to do occasional physical exams, and she would have to be competent when faced with the task.

It was with relief and a sense of humility that she moved on to her specialty training in psychiatry. At least in psychiatry, she thought, you can spend time with patients. Precious time. You don't get diverted by all that biological disease.

The first year of psychiatric training required considerable adjustment: going from a world of stethoscopes, cardiograms, flesh, bodily fluids, and numbers on laboratory slips to a world where words—their perception, interpretation, and manipulation—were her chief stock-in-trade.

"My God," she said to me after the first year. "I've never spent so much time just plain listening in my whole life." For a talkative person like Sallie, there was agony in learning to remain silent, letting the patient tell the story without intrusion. Again and again, her supervisors would tell her: "You were talking too much. You have to learn to be patient. Learn to take time. Give the patient the opportunity to trust you." Sallie wasn't even sure that trust was a reasonable expectation. Why should patients trust her? She was an awkward amateur. No matter how much she wanted to be of help, she had little assurance that her performance matched her desires.

But gradually Sallie became a more self-confident listener. She could listen for hours on end, hearing not only the words but the meaning behind the words. She learned to ask questions in new ways, to turn events this way and that, and to look at them from all sides.

And the stories she heard! She wouldn't have believed that there could be so much pain and suffering in so many ordinary-appearing people. Complete strangers would come to her and immediately start telling her the most intimate details of extraordinarily complex inner lives. First Sallie felt a sense of awe and privilege, tinged with guilt, at the voyeuristic opportunities extended to her by her new vocation. She dreamed that she was a thrush in an acacia tree, observing from above the private entanglements of lovers in an isolated field.

The metaphor was apt in many ways, for despite her own experiences and her undergraduate expectations, she found herself viewing patients from a measured distance. She was a professional. It was not her business to become embroiled in the private lives of her patients. They had come to her for expert help. An expert needed to have reliable dispassion, to be able to perform an objective assessment of relevant data, and to intervene without the distraction of self-interest.

Yet her task was to go beyond observing and listening. She was there to help. But how? What could she do? She was struck by the incongruousness of the situation: she, a young and relatively inexperienced student, seeking to guide and counsel persons half again her age, sometimes twice her age, who had lived lives sometimes beyond her ability to comprehend.

She was grateful to those patients who seemed to feel better just talking to her. It felt good to be of assistance, even though she was unsure exactly what she had done that could be considered helpful. The ones who did not get better simply by talking presented more of a challenge. These more difficult patients were the reason for all her training, she was told. The ones who could get better simply by ventilating could be talking to practically any decent and receptive person, with or without training.

Sallie started her second year of psychiatric training on an in-patient unit; she was assigned to be a resident psychiatrist on a ward in one of the university's teaching hospitals. This particular ward was designated as a drug-rehabilitation unit for addicts—and, in retrospect, Sallie thinks it was a terrible place for psychiatric training. Terrible because of what it did to her perception of patients, and terrible because of the way it eroded her sense of her own value as a physician and psychiatrist.

The ward itself contained twenty-six beds, hospitalese for a ward capacity of twenty-six patients. The beds, however, also symbolized a major irony, in that the patients themselves were in no way to be considered bedridden or physically incapacitated. On the contrary. To the extent that one can generalize about the patients she saw during her six-month stint on the ward, the typical patient was a male in his early twenties, with restless energy, sinewy strength, a keen eye toward personal survival, and a willingness to sleep anywhere so long as his sleep was facilitated by a drug of his own choosing, usually heroin, but sometimes barbiturates.

Most patients had arrest records, but one never knew for sure. They changed names and identities as required by the demands of the moment. Some were on probation from the court. Although the ward had a rule that no one could become a patient while under arrest or awaiting trial, it was common practice to find that patients already admitted to the ward had undisclosed charges pending against them. Most found that the courts would be more lenient with them if they could demonstrate that they had "voluntarily" sought treatment for their "disease," so it suited the addicts' purpose to be admitted to the hospital, and subterfuge seldom stood in their way.

Sallie was never sure when she could believe what her patients told her and when she could not. She felt intimidated by these streetwise young men, mostly her age or a few years younger yet so skilled in the art of survival in a hostile environment.

She wanted to have a doctor-patient relationship based on trust, but often that seemed impossible. It was apparent to everyone that many of the patients brought illicit drugs onto the wards or had their visitors do so. The situation was preposterous. It was frustrating to try to have any impact on the patients' drug dependence when the ward itself was a veritable marketplace for illegal drug activity. Those patients who really were motivated to quit drug use—and Sallie initially thought these constituted a majority—deserved better. They needed a haven away from the easy accessibility of hard drugs.

Sallie's initial impulse was to discharge all the patients she perceived as troublemakers, but it was difficult to differentiate the rogues from the near-rogues. What were to be her criteria? If she discharged all the people who, on casual observation, were found to be using drugs, she knew that she would fail to detect a number who also used drugs but did so surreptitiously. She would provide the facade of a drug-free ward, but not the reality. She would simply be punishing lack of stealth. Who was she to punish people, anyway? She was a doctor not a police officer.

If she discharged those who in confidence told her, their doctor, of personal drug use, she would be punishing honesty. If she searched all visitors and patients, and instituted a rigorous blood- and urine-test system to screen patients for illicit drug use, the place would feel like a prison and she would feel like a warden. Yet if she ignored the whole problem, she would fail to have achieved a therapeutic atmosphere in which motivated patients had a reasonable chance to overcome their habit.

Any medical treatment of addiction had to take into account the natural predilections of the patient population, and make compromises, but none of the compromises seemed satisfactory. Sallie asked her supervisors for guidance, but she heard no magic answers.

Sometimes she would sit quietly at the ward nursing station, staring reflectively at her charges. She tried to see them empathetically, to see them as victims of early life experiences and of extraordinary social forces. She tried to remember what it had been like for her when she, as a hospitalized psychiatric patient, had herself felt so victimized. She wanted so much to see herself as an ally of her patients.

Little things intruded. Several nurses had their purses stolen. At first all the patients denied any knowledge; but then when they were confronted, a dozen different stories emerged and it was impossible to tell which if any were true. Sallie's wallet was stolen from her purse when she left her office unguarded to resuscitate a patient who had overdosed. Several medical books, a stethoscope, and a blood-pressure cuff disappeared. Everything had to be locked up. There was no sense of trust whatsoever.

On one occasion a hospital security guard came upon two of her patients in a men's room near the hospital coffee shop. One was in the process of shooting up—injecting heroin into a vein in his forearm. The bathroom was filled with the acrid blue smoke of marijuana. The security guard reported the incident to the hospital administrator, who discussed the matter with Sallie and her supervisor.

When the two addicts were confronted, they adopted a pose of injured innocence. What was the fuss? they wanted to know. Even Sallie smoked marijuana on hospital grounds, the pair said. The charge wasn't true and it wasn't even relevant; but as a consequence, Sallie spent several long hours with the hospital authorities defending herself. It was an unpleasant task, made more awkward by the fact that one of the patients had overheard Sallie and a nurse discussing a staff party at which marijuana had been a part of the festivities.

The following day Sallie confronted all the patients on the ward with the blatant lies of two of its members. She was stunned when they were amused. They thought the pair had responded with adaptive creativity. When Sallie expressed her outrage, the ward occupants adopted a much more serious and disapproving manner—but Sallie disbelieved their sincerity. They were simply pretending, she sensed, to assuage her feelings and to protect themselves from her.

Her simmering frustration bubbled into controlled rage, and she lashed out at them: "I've always thought that trust was the cornerstone of a decent doctor-patient relationship. I tried to trust you, but I can't. Why should I? Any of you? You steal and you lie. You hurt people. You say one thing to my face and another to the nurses and a third to your fellow junkies. None of you trust one another. Why should I trust you?"

Yet how the hell could she presume to treat them as their doctor if she distrusted them? The problem of addiction seemed beyond her, and these patients were beyond her. They were indeed human beings, but so was she—and she had her limitations. Trusting them was like opening her home to a band of thieves. She couldn't do it. She would be emotionally ripped off again and again. The dilemma was too big for Sallie, and she felt herself starting to flee emotionally. She remained physically on the ward, but her heart wasn't in it.

She understood that the patients saw themselves as having no viable, attractive alternative to drugs, and she understood the powerful anodyne that heroin provided; but she couldn't identify with them at all. Every time she was in their presence, she felt herself becoming more judgmental—and self-righteous as well.

She wanted to respect her patients as human beings, but how can you respect people whose values you abhor? How could she, who had chosen to become a healer, form therapeutic alliances with people whose whole lives were pictures of self-destruction?

These were bad people, she thought, with no ethical sense whatsoever. She didn't think of them as sick, or label them with psychopathologic diagnoses. In her mind they were crooks and punks, with occasional redeeming features—but not enough in the aggregate to be worth her time.

Sallie endured her six months on the drug-treatment unit. She may have helped some of her patients, but she has no confidence that she did. Patients thanked her for her kindness and assistance, but she gave no credence to their words.

At the end of the six months, Sallie moved to another of the university's teaching hospitals, where she was to be a resident on a more traditional psychiatric ward. But she had become a different person. Where she had entered medical school skeptical of persons in authority, and a fierce partisan of patients, she was now as skeptical of her patients as she was of her professors. The imprimatur of patienthood by no means automatically conferred virtue on persons seeking medical care. But she couldn't yet call her cynicism by its true name. Her fall from grace had been too swift.

"I've just gotten realistic, that's all," she says. "My potential contribution to patients comes from my ability to apply the medical and psychiatric knowledge that I have worked hard to master. I'll try to maintain a humanistic perspective, to be respectful of my patients, but I'm not going to trust them automatically, and I'm not going to give them my heart automatically. I'm beginning to learn that compassion not only isn't always helpful, but sometimes it's counterproductive. It makes me vulnerable, and robs me of the energy to do what my medical training has prepared me to do. Any patient who wants compassion and trust from me has got to earn it."

7 THE DOCTOR-PATIENT RELATIONSHIP: In Pursuit of Integration

Like Sallie, most students begin the third year of medical school—when they first start to have extensive patient contact—with abundant energy for compassionate, sensitive, and respectful care of patients. More often than not, they are critical of the crassness they see in older physicians, and express their views in a manner which ranges from gentle reproach to diatribe. We respond in turn with varying degrees of defensiveness and hostility. It's hard to contest their values, and we remember with bittersweet nostalgia the hope we once had for changing the system, and of being idealized, lovable, kindly, and technically competent practitioners.

As the students begin to understand the futility of attempting to know all and do all there is to do, and of trying to provide truly comprehensive, integrated, and ideal health care, most of them set limits for themselves. The traditional way doctors have chosen to limit their responsibilities to patients has been through specialization. By focusing on the eyes or the urinary tract, a physician specialist can maintain reasonable levels of technical competence in one particular area—but at the expense of ignoring or slighting the rest of the body and the rest of the person.

That was part of my own rationale for becoming a psychiatrist; I found I couldn't do it all, so I decided to concentrate on that portion of medicine which was of greatest interest to me. The process actually began before medical school, though I understood little of it at the time.

I became a doctor for a variety of reasons, most of them relatively unconscious at the time. Motivation toward choosing a career can be difficult to sort out. The fact that my father was a physician certainly played an important role, as did my mother's often stated belief that there was no finer profession than medicine. She had always regretted that she herself had not studied medicine.

I think my own aspirations focused upon what I perceived as the essential nobility of the profession. I believed that the work would promote the best in me that I had to give, that it would help me become the kind of person that I wanted to be. I thought that in becoming a physician, I would be respected—because the profession was worthy of respect, and because I would be worthy of respect too.

When I entered medical school, I had vague intentions of becoming a city version of a country general practitioner. Gradually, as I was exposed to the avalanche of facts which constitutes medical training, I began to feel that I wasn't smart or hardworking enough to be a good general practitioner. It seemed to me that a conscientious GP was doomed to a lifetime of feeling intellectually inadequate, emotionally drained, and physically exhausted. In my third year I began to look around for a suitable specialty choice. I thought about specialties as diverse as ophthalmology (my father's specialty), gastroenterology, and public health. I did not consciously consider psychiatry.

But personal factors—and pure chance—nudged me toward my future. I was at that time living in my parents' home in Omaha. My father was becoming increasingly disabled from multiple sclerosis, with deteriorating coordination, bowel and bladder control, and intellectual function. My mother was struggling to attend to my father and sixteen-year-old sister, holding down two jobs, torn by her fidelity to her domestic responsibilities on the one hand and, on the other, her desperate desire to flee from a fate that was grinding all vitality and hope out of her.

Those were difficult years for all of us: my mother tense and demanding, intermittently erupting with frustrated rage; my sister dutiful and unhappy, struggling through an awkward adolescence; and my father, loneliest of us all, sitting endlessly in front of the TV set, watching everything and remembering nothing, as all the connections in his neurological system gradually deteriorated within him.

It's hard for me to say what I was like during that time, not because the recollection is so painful but because I had erected so sturdy a facade that my real feelings were hidden even from myself. I was responsible, holding down several jobs all through medical school because my family had no financial reserves. I was self-sufficient, making no emotional demands on my family because they had no emotional reserves. I was amiable and cheerful, a family peacemaker, an entertainer and compromiser. Many of my Omaha friends thought me critical and occasionally biting, but I didn't really acknowledge those qualities in myself until much later.

In the winter of my third year of medical school I took my required training in psychiatry and had the good fortune to have a wonderfully talented teacher as my immediate supervisor. Dr. Margaret Peterson helped me to understand and accept my own feelings in a way that I had never done before. It was the beginning of a process that has continued ever since. She helped me to discover that my primary interest in medicine was the emotional effect of disease on the person in which it resided, on the family, and on all other persons affected by the process.

I decided to go into psychiatry, for it seemed to be the best path, both to help me in my own attempts at personal discovery and because no other area of medicine focused so deliberately on the struggles of human beings attempting to cope with the disruption of disease. If family practice had been a formal specialty at that time, with accompanying residency training and specialty board certification, I might have chosen that path; but it wasn't. Family practice didn't achieve formal specialty status until 1969.

I graduated from medical school in 1966 and took a rotating internship at the University of Pennsylvania Graduate Hospital in Philadelphia. A "rotating internship" designates a year that provides a little bit of advanced training in all the principal areas of medical care—surgery, pediatrics, obstetrics, and internal medicine. I chose that course both because I still harbored some wish to be a well-rounded general practitioner and because I knew I would be going into military service for two years. It was the Vietnam era, and male physicians had to perform their two-year selective service obligation.

I spent the next two years as a general medical officer in the Coast

Guard, on an icebreaker in the Arctic, on a cargo transport in the western Pacific, and at Coast Guard bases in Yorktown, Virginia; Cape May, New Jersey; Governors Island, New York; and Alameda, California. When I was aboard ship, for as long as five months at a time, I was often the only physician for thousands of miles in any direction. Under those circumstances, I earned the title that my medical degree had supposedly conferred upon me a couple of years before: I became a doctor, someone capable—more or less—of assuming responsibility for the lives and health of several hundred persons.

The irony is that I got so much ego satisfaction from doing so little. There were approximately two hundred men aboard each of the ships on which I served, all of them in abundantly good health, and the occasional injuries or disorders from which they suffered could have, with rare exceptions, been as well cared for by the corpsman as by myself. Yet the men aboard the two ships on which I served treated me with a touching deference. In the event of disease or disaster, I was their link with life. I was their doctor. They treated me with respect, not simply because of my presumed skills, which they were poorly equipped to judge, but because I was responsible for them— and they perceived that I took that responsibility seriously.

After the service, I entered my residency in psychiatry at Stanford. Under the Stanford umbrella, I had a broad range of clinical experience at the Stanford University Medical Center itself, at the Palo Alto Veterans Administration Hospital, at the San Mateo County Hospital, and at the Royal Edinburgh Hospital in Scotland. From Stanford I went to practice and to teach as a psychiatrist in San Francisco. I've been teaching medical students at the University of California at San Francisco—sometimes on a salaried basis and sometimes on a nonsalaried volunteer basis—since 1972.

My first job was at the San Francisco Veterans Administration Hospital, one of the principal teaching hospitals of UCSF, where I chose to work in part because they had a good job open for me, but also because I felt I owed the V. A. a debt. My father was, and is, a totally disabled veteran. My sister had gone through college with the help of my father's V. A. benefits. Without the help of the V. A., and some professional courtesy from my father's physician colleagues, my family would have been financially devastated by the medical bills incurred by both my parents' medical ailments, and by my father's decade-long stay in a nursing home. I believed deeply that traditional fee-for-service medical practice tended to rob American families of their financial health, even as it restored the patient's physical health.

At the V. A., I worked as a psychotherapist, and first worked on and then directed the psychiatric consultation service of the large general hospital. My job was to provide psychiatric consultations to physicians in other specialties who were struggling with some aspect of patient care in which someone with my background and interest might provide useful advice. The consultation generally focused on one of three types of problems: diagnosis, treatment, or management.

The diagnostic problems typically called for me to assist in the process of labeling patients in a useful manner. For instance: "This patient who just had a heart attack is behaving strangely; what is the explanation or diagnosis?" Or: "This patient with chronic diarrhea isn't getting any better; to what degree are psychological factors contributory, and what are they?"

The treatment problems were a natural corollary to the diagnostic ones: "Please help us treat this patient who is acutely depressed over the impending amputation of her lower leg." Or: "This patient has hysterical blindness; can you help us help him regain his vision?"

The management consultations were more amorphous and less obviously related to technical knowledge and skills. They concerned patients who wouldn't take medicine as directed, or who were planning on leaving the hospital against medical advice, or who were seen as inappropriately critical of the staff. Occasionally, the questions would focus on the staff itself: "We've had six deaths on the ward in the past two weeks; we're all depressed as hell; can you help us put things in a more useful perspective?"

In response to these three categories of consultations—and some other more infrequent ones—I regularly gave advice and guidance, and did my best to teach students, house officers, nurses, and others to give more psychologically sophisticated care, so that they could take care of patients' minds and bodies in an integrated fashion.

No matter how much time and energy I put into this task, it was apparent that the lessons I taught were seldom incorporated into a given physician's ongoing repertoire of skills. Again and again, the physicians ran into the same sets of problems because they did not take time to get to know their patients as human beings, did not investigate personal and social factors related to the patients' care, and did not allow themselves to engage in a reciprocal, collaborative relationship with their patients.

As I pondered my inability to alter the behavior of my students, I of course first blamed them for being refractory to my teaching. They were narrow, insensitive, and too insecure to attempt new strategies in dealing with patients.

That was purely defensive, a rationalization on my part. All my personal experiences with students in seminars and social occasions contradicts these assumptions. To be sure, there are some crass students, but the majority start off just as we might wish. It is the role they assume that changes them.

Suddenly it dawned on me: here I was teaching the students about the psyche and asking them to integrate that information with the care of the patients' physical health, while I was blissfully free of any such responsibility myself. I was responsible only for the psyche. Was there anyone around who successfully provided both high-quality treatment of disease and high-quality care of the patient as a person?

The medical school where I taught, and still teach, is prestigious, often ranked among the top ten in the country by pollsters who think such surveys are meaningful. I started to ask the students: "Who are the master clinicians on the faculty? People whose clinical skill and human understanding of patients constitute role models for yourself?" The students used to name three individuals regularly out of a faculty of several thousand, but two of the three—one man and one woman—have since moved elsewhere. Now there is only one left, and he does no research and is worried that he won't be awarded tenure.

I also asked the students, "Who on the psychiatry faculty understands human beings, how they function in health and illness, and can apply that knowledge in a way that you want to emulate yourself?" They looked at me blankly in return. This professor knows everything about marijuana research, and that one is an expert on tricyclic antidepressants, but a role model in humanity . . . ? There are none.

The students often think, but seldom say, that it's too easy to preach about integrating the art and science of medicine and too hard to practice it. The internists and surgeons talk about the technical aspects of disease and its treatment but seldom devote time to psychological issues. Those few who do are rarely able to practice what they preach. The psychiatrists and social scientists focus on the psychosocial issues, but almost never devote time and energy to the diagnosis and treatment of physical disease. Everybody talks about integration of psyche and soma, but—until they give up—the only people who are still trying to accomplish integration are the students; and they end up feeling like chumps for trying.

That was one of the principal reasons that I decided to give general practice a try again. I wanted to see if I—a fully trained and board-certified psychiatrist—could practice general medicine and still retain the kind of sensitivity I had been demanding of my students.

Now when I talk to the students about integration of art and science, my words carry some authenticity—but I make no pretense of being a paragon for them to mold themselves after. I'm struggling, I tell the students. I have my successes, but humility overwhelms pride. I save myself from total exhaustion only by constantly making compromises, and accepting my limits and those of the system in which I work.

I teach in a different setting now, though still at the same school. I meet with students in small groups on a weekly basis to discuss psychological aspects of medical practice, and to focus on practical means for enhancing their functioning as human beings in the doctor-patient relationship.

The series of classes began as a pilot project at the University of California at San Francisco Medical Center in 1977, and I became part of it the following year. I'm one of a faculty of thirty or so. For two hours each week, the students meet with one of us to discuss psychiatric aspects of patient care in the various hospital wards and clinics where the students are assigned: surgery, medicine, neurology, obstetrics, and so forth. We interview patients, talk about practical aspects of the doctor-patient relationship, and try to suggest useful strategies for coping with human problems in medical care. Generally, those we treat aren't psychiatric patients; they're just ordinary people struggling with illness and the process of treatment.

When the classes go well, especially at the beginning of each year, the students work hard to understand illness and the process of hospitalization from the patient's standpoint. I try to help them use what they hear in a constructive way, so that they can be full human beings with their patients, not simply technicians on the one hand or so idealistically giving on the other that they become unable to sustain their commitment to sensitive and personalized patient care. But in the face of all the forces pushing the students in other directions, the classes are like the tail trying to wag the dog.

On a recent occasion I met with a group of eight students, five men and three women, during their first eight weeks of patient care. They were a particularly good group: verbal, sensitive, bright, well intentioned, mature, with considerable background in social sciences and the humanities. I can't imagine a randomly picked group of medical students more likely to be receptive to the kinds of things our seminar was designed to teach.

Yet over the first eight weeks of clinical experience, the growth of cynicism was astounding. Patients who at first were called Mr. Smith and Miss Jones at best became "the case of pancreatitis" or "my diabetic in room two thirty-eight." Many patients were referred to as "turkeys" and "gomers" or perceived as leeches who sucked from the students more compassion than they had to give.

The students listen seriously to what I have to say. Many are grateful for the classes, grateful for time away from their other responsibilities, time devoted to reflection and nurturance of humanistic values in medicine. But overall, their attitude—especially as the junior year progresses—is best described as leery. They look around them and perceive that even the stresses of medical school are only a foreshadowing of the multitude of pressures that they will feel in the future, pressures that separate physicians from their ideals and cause patients to resent their doctors.

The students sense these things, and they begin to move cautiously. They begin to wonder what kinds of compromises they will choose for themselves, and how much of the choice will be up to them.

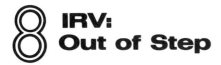

IRV:
Out of Step

If you saw Irv walking to his car at the end of the day, you might think that he was working too hard. Shoulders hunched forward, eyes fixed upon the ground, skin pastelike, gait labored, shoes squeaking, he looks as if he's carrying the world's burdens on the nape of his neck. If you saw him first thing in the morning, he would look no different. Irv has been putting one foot before the other for years.

People who work with Irv often remark on how much he looks like his patients, most of whom are men in advancing middle age, military veterans of World War II and Korea, who to all outward assessment appear whupped by life. Irv attracts such patients by the hundreds, and the affinity between doctor and patients often defies the understanding of interested onlookers.

If you were to arrive on an average afternoon at the Veterans Administration clinic where Irv works, you would see a room filled with men waiting patiently to see their psychiatrist. Occasionally they exchange small talk, but mostly they sit in silence. Periodically, one will hear his name called, go to Irv's office, spend ten to fifteen minutes there, and emerge carrying a prescription. Some come weekly, some monthly, and some irregularly.

Younger psychiatrists who work in the clinic tend to deprecate

Irv's clinical acumen and therapeutic style. He prescribes too much medicine, they say. He processes people. He talks too much and listens too little, has no in-depth understanding of what goes on in his patients' unconscious.

If you were to ask Irv's patients what they think of him, the picture would be far more positive. "Aw, he's okay," one says. "He understands me," says another. "He cares." Over and over again, from a group of generally not very articulate men, the sense that emerges is one of great fondness and loyalty—and of a relationship between doctor and patient that is sustaining in a way the patients are hard put to describe.

I remember standing outside Irv's office on one occasion, eavesdropping on the sounds audible through the porous government-issue door. The patient who had just entered the office was pathetic in appearance: a man with a mashed-potato face covered with beard stubble, wearing two overcoats, a shirt with missing buttons, frayed and baggy trousers, and mildewed shoes with trailing laces. In the waiting room, the man had been carrying on a spirited conversation with some unseen presence, vigorously gesticulating all the while.

As soon as he walked into the office, Irv launched into him.

"Goddamn it, Sergeant, look at you! You are a mess, a miserable goddamn mess! Aren't you?"

Silence.

"Aren't you?" The inflection adding a note of command.

More silence.

"Answer me, goddamn it!" Irv's fist pounds his desk top, and the door between us rattles. "Are you or are you not a mess?"

"Yessir," comes a soft reply.

"Yessir what?" demands Irv.

"Yessir, I'm a mess."

"And you are starting to hear voices again, aren't you?"

"Yessir, I am."

"And you are starting to act crazy as a loon again, and everybody stares at you and thinks you are an A-number-one loony again, don't they?"

"Yessir, they do."

"And you haven't been eating well or getting out of your hotel room, have you?"

"No sir, I haven't."

"And it's all because you stopped taking your medications again, isn't it?"

"Yessir, but . . ."

"Goddamn it, Sergeant," Irv roars. "I don't want to hear your excuses. You always have excuses when you stop taking your pills. What I want to see is some performance. I'm giving you a simple order and I want you to carry it out. Is that asking too much?"

"No sir."

"Okay, I'm writing out this prescription, and I want you to get it filled and I want you to take the medication as it tells you to on the label. Is that understood?"

"Yessir, I understand."

"And I want to see you here next week, at the same time. Is that understood?"

"Yessir, I'll be here."

"And when I see you, I want you to be shaved, I want to see buttons on your shirt, and I want you looking like you take some pride in your appearance. You're a good-looking man when you make the effort."

"Yessir, I'll make the effort."

"And I want you to bring me a movie ticket stub to show me that you've gotten out of your hotel room, and I want to see a cash register receipt so I know that you've been buying yourself enough groceries. Okay?"

"Yessir. I'll do that."

"You're a good man, Sergeant. I'll see you next week."

"Yessir."

After Irv's patient shuffled out, I went in and sat down and accepted a mug of instant coffee, thrust at me without comment.

"Tell me about the sergeant, Irv."

"Yalu River," Irv says.

Despite Irv's relative loquaciousness with his patients, he is not much of a conversationalist. He listens for a living, and gets his fill of it with his patients. When a sociable sentence looks as though it's going to become a paragraph, Irv starts getting restless.

The last thing he wants to hear when he is away from patients are people's troubles. Not from acquaintances, not from co-workers, not from anyone. He's heard so many troubles in his life that they sprinkle his shoulders like so much dandruff.

When I want to chat with someone, there's no sense going to see Irv. Irv communicates telegraphically, sputtering out a few phrases at a time. To someone who doesn't know him, his code words often seem strange and out of place. Is the man crazy?

To someone who does know Irv, the words *Yalu River* convey volumes of meaning, placing the sergeant as a person whose life is consistent with Irv's view on the nature of existence. To Irv, life is a process of retreat and the patching up of wounds. Retreat from aspirations and retreat from illusions. Wounds of the body and wounds of the spirit. Fortunate people retreat in an orderly fashion, tending to their wounds as they go; the unfortunate retreat blindly, erratically, agonizingly, the wounds open for all to see.

Irv was a general medical officer, not yet a psychiatrist, performing his selective service obligation in a field hospital in the early days of the Korean War. Irv remembers November 24, 1950, with icy clarity. On that day, MacArthur launched his Yalu offensive and assured reporters and his own troops that the war would come to an end shortly.

Two days later, thirty-three Chinese divisions hit the United Nations line, and Irv's battalion caught the full impact. Every night the enemy flares lit up the sky, their eerie trumpets and clanging cymbals sounding a terrifying warning, and then the masses of Chinese troops would come at them out of the darkness in wave after wave. No matter how many enemy were killed, it made no difference. Irv's battalion was surrounded, suffocated by the enemy. The frozen, rocky ground offered no shelter. The frigid, cutting air brought only terror, dismemberment, and death.

Irv and the rest of the hospital staff did what they could, holding remnants of lives together while the field hospital around them collapsed in preparation for the day's retreat and reassembled in the evening in preparation for the night's attack. Sometimes they didn't have time to reassemble the hospital. Sometimes they operated on the back of a canvas-covered truckbed. The steel decking would become so slippery with blood and other body materials that the surgeons risked slipping when they shifted their weight from one tired foot to another. Fatigue permeated existence, displaced all sensibility, even the horror of battle. Everything was ragged: the retreat, the soldiers' bodies, the souls of the survivors. The only salvation to those terrible days was the comradeship of men under fire, the exquisite moments of loyalty and caring from men who had nothing else to give and no reason to give anything except the knowledge of their shared humanity, which miraculously had not abandoned them altogether.

After the war Irv decided to go into psychiatry. He never again wanted to see inside another chest or abdomen, and he decided that he needed psychiatric help himself. He was barely holding on to his own sanity, and thought that in the process of studying psychiatry he might learn enough to put together the pieces in his own head. Each night he had nightmares: garish, violent dreams from which he would awaken drenched in chilling sweat and with the sickening memory of the sweet deadly aroma of gangrene.

Early on, he gravitated to the Veterans Administration, choosing to spend the rest of his professional life with men and women who had been in the armed forces. When he looks at his patients he sees battle scars, masses of battle scars, even where a casual observer would see none. As Irv has aged, his therapeutic style has become increasingly idiosyncratic. He follows his instincts and cares little for the dictates of others who try to define what constitutes quality care.

"Do you think what you do with the sergeant can be called psychotherapy?" I ask.

"What does it matter?" he responds.

"Do you think what you do helps him?"

"Probably," he says. "Sometimes yes, sometimes no. I don't know anything else that would work any better."

Irv has been seeing the sergeant as an outpatient at intervals for almost fifteen years. The sergeant lives in a single room in a residential hotel occupied almost exclusively by pensioners. He lives alone with his memories and his dreams, and they sometimes become so real to him that the boundary of fantasy melts away and he is unable to distinguish between apparitions and the pedestrian demands of life. Irv believes, probably correctly, that the sergeant would have been hospitalized repeatedly if he had been seeing almost any other psychiatrist, but Irv manages to keep him out of the asylum. Somehow the commanding officer charade they go through together keeps the sergeant from deteriorating completely.

Irv participates in bizarre charades with many of his patients, and it often makes him look pretty peculiar to outsiders. He doesn't worry about it. You can't spend an entire professional life working with madmen and not become a little mad yourself. He accepts his eccentricities as professional equipment. Even the term *madmen* has little meaning for him.

Is the sergeant crazy? Irv won't answer the question. He waves it away. The sergeant's just a human being. One has to expect peculiarities in human beings. The labels mean nothing. Worse, they are stigmatizing. Let other people label patients with pseudodiagnostic tags. He wants none of it.

"What did you write in the chart?" I ask Irv. He shoves the medical record across the desk for me to see. The entry for this date reads simply, "Routine visit, Rx Stelazine."

"That will never pass chart review," I say.

Irv gives me a look of disdain. His clinic, in an effort to monitor quality of medical care, has begun to actively review all patients' charts to make sure that they conform to standard. Each entry should include the patient's statement of the reason for the visit, the doctor's objective findings, the doctor's assessment, and a clear description of what was done.

Irv hates it. "If the record is good enough to be approved by the committee," he says, "it's too good to be handed over."

He could rub it in a bit, but he doesn't. In 1973, I wrote an embarrassingly messianic article about quality control in psychiatry—about how important it was and how it could be achieved by more diligent medical record-keeping. It took me a while to realize how naïve and simplistic I had been. Irv took a satisfied relish in watching my maturation.

I still write more in the patient's medical record than Irv does, but considerably less than I used to. The increasing conciseness of my prose in medical records is not a consequence of laziness. Rather, I feel that the intricacies patients tell me about their personal lives are no one's business but theirs and mine, and certainly not the business of persons who review hospital charts for completeness.

The preliminary chart reviews are performed by junior clerks in the medical records office. They have a primer introduction to medical terminology and no formal professional training, and it's foolish to assume that they can be held to professional standards of confidentiality. To put in writing the details of the sergeant's experiences and feelings would be to submit them to the avid eyes of youngsters in their late adolescence. All the patients Irv sees have stories to tell. All of them have personal histories that could provide material for snick-

ering gossip, or for pulpy tales in sordid magazines, or even for black-
mail. It smacks of betrayal to expose the confidential details of private lives to hospital file clerks.

Irv is incensed at the tendency in medicine to judge a physician's
performance by what he or she puts in the chart. All too often, such
emphasis merely encourages the physician to spend precious minutes
writing justifications for what was or was not done, instead of spending the same amount of time with the patients.

Not only do "quality-control requirements" mandate chart completeness, but so do the evidentiary requirements of the law. If Irv
were to testify in the courtroom—for example, if one of his patients
were involved in judicial proceedings or if Irv were somehow sued for
malpractice—any decent prosecuting attorney could make him appear to be an incompetent. The chart as a document gives no evidence of the time and caring and skill that Irv brings to his patients,
nor does it offer proof of how much he knows about them.

Actually, given his individualistic style, he may be correct in thinking that he is better off leaving the chart nearly empty. He says of the
quality-control committee at his clinic: "If I put down what I actually
do, they would think me even more of a circus clown than they do
already."

I shake my head in sympathy. Poor Irv. Everybody likes to be appreciated, and it's clear that he doesn't feel very much appreciated at
all.

"Do they let you get away with such skimpy notes?" I ask.

"The chart review committee put me on probation," he says, with
one of his rare grins. "But if they get rid of me, they'll have to find
someone to see all my patients."

Irv sees all the patients no one else wants to see. The lost souls. The
forgotten men. The dirty and uriniferous. The people who come year
after year, rarely speaking a word. Hopeless shadows, with never anything exciting or clever to say. Almost all of them are chronic patients, expecting no cure, unlikely to show dramatic changes. Like
most physicians, Irv has seen his practice age along with him. When
he started, he treated mostly men and women in their twenties and
thirties, people for whom the clock ticked slowly and for whom the
passage of time signaled at least some hope. Now the majority are in
their fifties and sixties, and some in their seventies, and not a season
goes by without some deaths among them—most by natural causes

and occasionally one by suicide. Irv has been through it all dozens of times. He is a chronic therapist and his work holds no surprises for him any more.

"Don't you ever get discouraged, Irv?" I ask.

He stares at me for what seems like minutes, with the saddest eyes imaginable, the barest hint of another smile on his lips.

"I'm sorry," I say. "It was a stupid question." Irv's always discouraged. Discouragement is the hallmark of a life spent among an army in retreat. Irv expects nothing beyond the occasional satisfaction he gets from the wounded he meets along the way. We are all battle casualties, he believes. The only difference is our level of awareness, our concern for our fellows.

On Irv's desk is a simply framed picture of his wife and fifteen-year-old son. I know them: quiet, somber people, just like Irv. How could it be otherwise? Irv with a sprightly wife and child seems unimaginable to me, just as I've always taken it for granted that he would never have his morning eggs sunny-side up.

I've seen the three of them walking arm in arm through the park. What does this man bring home to them from his work? I wonder. Who brings the cheerfulness into their home? Surely not Irv. What will the son be like, with a father whose view of humanity stems from daily contact with the bruised and hopeless? What does Irv get from them which fuels him to spend his professional life among the walking wounded?

But Irv seems happy with his family—or at least what passes for happy with him.

His only real bitterness comes when he reflects on his status within his profession. The work he does is commonly regarded as drudge work, and many see Irv as a bit of a drudge himself. Irv's method with patients, though derived from years of work as a clinician, has an intuitive, seat-of-the-pants style to it—and Irv has a difficult time explaining and justifying it to quality-care review committees.

How does one measure the value of what Irv does? By giving him a multiple-choice exam and counting up the score? By looking over his collection of patients and seeing how many "cures" he has achieved? By asking for testimonials from patients or colleagues? How would one select which patients and colleagues to ask? Irv is a man with many detractors. He falls short by many measures.

One group of patients with whom Irv gets along poorly are angry young men with fervent illusions of how life and the world ought to be. Passionate, intrusive idealists, Irv calls them. He sees nothing ahead for such people but bitterness and eventual defeat. Something in him snaps, and he loses all patience. "Fools!" he'll mutter to himself, and he'll seek to flee from their presence.

On one occasion, Irv was spending his mandatory half-day per week covering the walk-in clinic for psychiatric emergencies. All psychiatrists in the clinic do this in rotation. A twenty-two-year-old veteran was brought in by three bigger and more muscular friends. He had become despondent over the loss of a girl friend and had raged around his apartment breaking everything in sight. His friends were concerned that he might hurt someone. He repeatedly vowed that if he could find his former girl friend he would kill her, as well as anyone else who got in his way. In the examining area, the young man overflowed with fury. He called his friends venomous names. He insulted the nurses and even spat at Irv. "I don't need no goddamn psychiatrist," he shouted. "I just want to kill the bitch."

Irv could see beyond the patient's rage, and see his hurt. He could understand that the aggressive behavior was in many ways an adaptive response to a devastating blow the patient had received to his own sense of self, and that some of his values and beliefs had been destroyed along with his previous loving relationship. Irv could see that, and he knew how to get to the young man's hurt. He knew the insistent words, the patient and soothing manner that might well change the young man's abrasive bravado to tears and shamed apologies.

He knew what could be done, but he had no patience for it. No taste for it. He turned on his heels and told the nurses: "Call the cops and tell them we've got a threatening homicidal person here. This isn't a medical problem."

Irv was technically correct, but his attitude upset a lot of people. Many staff people felt that he gave up too easily, that more could have been done. The young man's friends felt betrayed; they had brought the patient in good faith to a psychiatric facility for treatment, only to have him end up in jail. They ultimately wrote letters to the V. A. administrators, to various veterans' groups, and even one to a congressman requesting an investigation. To outward appearances, Irv withstood the commotion stoically. "Everyone gets along with some people better than others," he would say. "That's human enough. Surely you don't begrudge my being human every now and then."

Internally he found the stress considerable. His ulcer became a problem again, and he had to increase his medication and eat only tasteless, bland foods. Irv is terrified of having another massive gastro-intestinal hemorrhage. That last one was bad enough.

Irv feels little security in his job. It would be difficult to fire him, and the truth is that he is unlikely to be fired, but that doesn't keep him from worrying. He knows he works in hostile territory, but he feels too old to move elsewhere. He only has four years to go until retirement. Recently, a new director was brought in from outside to "upgrade" the clinic, which means—among other things—to get rid of Irv and people like him who lack board certification and who aren't abreast of the latest scientific developments.

The new director is a bright man, thoughtful and well meaning; but he has priorities that differ from Irv's in important respects. The new man values ideas and theories—and their informed discussion. He has done a great deal of research in brain chemistry and expects his staff to know all about such things. Irv knows he can't pass muster on very technical, scientific topics. Moreover, it's difficult for him to work up much enthusiasm for them.

"Theories are okay, for beginners," he says. "They give you something to hold onto until you work up some clinical common sense, but an old warhorse like me doesn't need to know all that. The theories are not only useless, they're confusing, and make me doubt the usefulness of the things I already know to be helpful. They make me less effective, not more effective. Among all the bright young science types, I'm a nothing, a relic of the pretechnologic age, a borderline incompetent."

The irony is that when Irv first entered psychiatry in the mid-1950s, he was one of the most progressive clinicians in his area. He was among the first to start using the major tranquilizers when they became available. He was an early participant in the group-theory movement, and for a long time he was one of the only psychiatrists in his city to actually make visits to his patients' homes. It was impossible for him to sustain that level of innovativeness and emotional commitment for twenty-five years, however. The work consumed him, and now he does what he can do, without berating himself for what he cannot. He takes care of patients one at a time, in brief visits, because he has no emotional reserves left.

"Shouldn't that be enough?" he asks, knowing that reality isn't simply a matter of "shoulds." He has not taken his specialty board exams and won't. He feels too old to study all that physiology and biochemistry and neuroanatomy all over again—and he doubts that it would alter his treatment of patients significantly. The subject prompts a rare monologue from him: "All the clinical research depresses me," says Irv. "The academic researchers crank out theories about new chemicals which may cause mental illness and new tests for this or that, and then to bolster their own sense of worth, to reassure themselves that what they do is important, they make us learn that stuff. They test us on specialty certification exams, which they run, and charge us money so they can lecture to us about it at continuing education seminars, which are required for relicensure. You go to continuing education seminars and they talk about things like 5-hydroxytryptamine and dihydroindole acetic acid. I'm not interested in that, and it has no relevance to my care of patients. It's not why I went into psychiatry. But we have to learn that crap because the profession won't float on compassion and sensitive listening alone. Science is pushing all the art in our profession to the sidelines. Before too long, there won't be any room in psychiatry and medicine for people like me."

Irv is bitter; and, in my less charitable moments, I tend to consider his observations and complaints as sour grapes, the cranky irritability of a lazy person who is stuck in patterns of behavior that no longer work, yet who lacks the gumption to make necessary changes.

Perhaps he's like a tired old plowhorse who curses tractors. Maybe there's nothing more to him than that. Yet it is precisely the plowhorse quality about him that I like, the countrified idiosyncratic wisdom that understands things that are not capable of being measured, and whose value can't be computed simply by looking up the age and model in a blue book.

Sometimes I look at Irv and wonder, Will I be outmoded too when I reach his age? How will our society be measuring the value of individual physicians in another twenty years?

9 THE DOCTOR-PATIENT RELATIONSHIP: Documenting Competence

Like most physicians, before I entered medical school I took it for granted that the doctor's primary function was to help people who were patients, not simply because doctors wished to do so, but because the nature of the work was intrinsically helpful. It was in the process of helping that I expected to find my own sense of worth and meaning in my professional life. It was in the process of assessing my helpfulness that I, or anyone else, could judge whether I was being a good doctor.

I still believe that I help some people, but not nearly as many as I would have imagined, and with most it's simply impossible for me or anyone else to know. Most doctors would share this uncertainty. We all face the issues of what we as physicians are trying to do with and for our patients. What is our central purpose? These questions are pressing because so many different parties behave as if they know the answers, and argue insistently for their special method of measuring our effectiveness in this way or that.

Irv thinks his main objective with the sergeant is to keep him out of the hospital. In his heart, he also believes that keeping the sergeant functioning—however marginally—for fifteen years outside the asylum constitutes a genuine accomplishment. Both he and the sergeant seem to believe that together they have done something of value, that the accomplishment is a joint one. Yet no one can prove that the sergeant would have been hospitalized had he not been seeing Irv, or even that the sergeant is necessarily better off for having stayed out of the hospital. Even if all this were true, were these accomplishments worth the cost?

Does it make sense to send someone like Irv through four years of college, four years of medical school, one year of internship, three years of psychiatric residency, so that the taxpayers can give him a handsome salary to keep the sergeant out of the asylum? Irv thinks so. The sergeant would probably feel too unworthy to vote on the issue, even if he could organize his thinking sufficiently to comprehend the question.

In the private practice settings of Chris and David, patients vote on their physicians with their own dollars and how they choose to use them. Times are changing, however, and private practice no longer dominates the medical-care picture. Increasingly the answers to such questions won't be formulated by the Irvs and the sergeants of this world. The doctors and their patients won't be the ones to vote—or, at least, their narrow opinions and feelings about one another won't determine the outcome. The issues are too big. They involve matters of access to health care, cost effectiveness, national priorities, and evolving techniques for measuring "health-care quality"—all vague and global considerations.

When Irv graduated from medical school in 1948, two-thirds of all physicians were in private practice, seeing patients whom they thought of as *their* patients, with a definite proprietary air. In turn, patients tended to be able to identify a physician as *their* physician, and to feel proprietary in turn. The nation at that time was just barely more metropolitan than not. It still had a rural and small-town flavor, and people believed they were able to judge the skills of those who provided them with services.

Now, well over half of all physicians go into salaried practice rather than private practice, and three-fourths of our nation's population lives in metropolitan areas. People don't know the doctors who treat them as well as they once did, are less likely to have an identifiable individual whom they refer to as their physician, and are less certain that they can judge accurately whether or not any given physician is an able practitioner.

The public now wants some external measure of the competence of the physicians from whom they seek care. Other factors have also led to the development of so-called quality-care measures: the rising cost of medical care and the growing role of third parties in financing it; the media's spotlighting of seemingly incompetent physicians who have escaped disciplinary procedures within their own ranks; and the escalating role of science and technology in medical care. Malpractice suits have added to these pressures. In California the average physician is now sued every four and a half years, and throughout the country the frequency and size of the settlements have more to do with geography and the physician's specialty than with any objective measures of quality of care.

Because of these multiple factors, and in part because of an "if-we-don't-do-it-ourselves-they'll-do-it-to-us" feeling, the medical profession has begun to develop techniques for assessing the quality of health care. The variety and diversity of these programs, as well as the stridency of their supporters and critics, suggests an uncomfortable conclusion: no one knows how to define quality of care, let alone measure it. One thing is certain, however. The measurement attempts will strive to use scientific methods and will focus on the definable, the measurable, and the documentable.

Psychiatry has been attempting to become more scientific and objective for at least a century, and there have been many events which have hastened the process. The postwar years have been the most dramatic in this regard. An explosion of interest in and funds for research followed World War II, a war won by the fruits of brilliant scientific investigation. All research in basic and applied science prospered, and the medical research community did very well indeed. Penicillin and streptomycin had just been discovered, and the miraculous cures of medicine's new wonder drugs created a mood of hope, and awed respect for medical scientists. Few would have disagreed with W. H. Auden when he said: "When I find myself in the company of scientists, I feel like a shabby curate who has strayed by mistake into a drawing room full of dukes." How alluring it was for bright young students to enter a scientific profession.

By the 1960s, while bright engineers were putting men on the moon and bright surgeons were transplanting organs, bright psychiatrists were measuring chemicals in the brain and organizing vast surveys plotting the psychological functioning of various "target" populations. The implications of all this activity, especially when it came time to ask for funding, was that in the end all these endeavors would pay for themselves: there would be therapeutic consequences that would lead to a better life for our people. The pleasant fiction assumed the magnitude of a shared delusion: money for research would always be well spent.

One of the largely unanticipated by-products of the scientific revolution in medicine and psychiatry is that being an artful clinician has gradually become a less prestigious and often less desirable goal for talented medical students than being a laboratory scientist. Spending time understanding patients as human beings somehow has come to seem less important, less rewarding, than time spent understanding laboratory tests. Medical-school faculty members remain predominantly research-oriented scientists—and administrators—rather than clinicians with sustained experience with individual patients.

Irv says he is a relic of a previous age, and in many ways he is. He has the bare minimum of credentials, and he resists all efforts to "update" his skills and document his ability. He thinks his most important therapeutic tool is himself and his humanity, and none of the quality-control devices know how to assess that. He thinks all the preoccupation with credentials and bits of paper to go on the wall is crap.

What kind of credentials should we and do we demand of our practitioners? All licensed physicians in this country are required to have a diploma from an approved medical school, which means approximately four years of education with requisite exposure to what are broadly accepted as "core" educational topics. Graduates of such programs are distinguished by three key qualities: measurable academic ability (as represented by performance on objective exams), endurance (as measured by attendance at required activities), and absence of blatantly reprehensible behavior. Subtleties of personal character—either positive or negative—tend to have little influence these days on whether or not a student passes. One can't quantify qualities like empathy or integrity, and professors are no longer allowed to make arbitrary subjective decisions. Students can sue if they are failed without solid objective cause.

After attaining the M. D. degree, there are two principal credentialing pathways, with some overlap between the two: the first involves specialty training and certification, and the second involves what is euphemistically called continuing medical education (CME).

Specialty training in this country is essentially an extension and narrowing of the medical-school experience. Trainees are asked to master incredible detail, and to assume ever greater responsibility in narrower and narrower aspects of patient care. While not all doctors who enter specialty training complete the process, the vast majority do. Those who don't, usually fail on grounds of inability to master technical detail or for lack of stamina. There is no evidence that trainees fail for inability to comprehend the subtleties of an idealized doctor-patient relationship.

The specialty certification exams are more of the same. To the limited extent that oral exams are included in the process in order to measure human qualities, there is no evidence to suggest that they are successful. In fact, there is considerable evidence to the contrary.

The American Board of Psychiatry and Neurology (ABPN), for example, currently gives a two-part examination, first written, then oral. The principal screening function is served by the multiple-choice written exam, which inevitably tests for mastery of technical data and quantifiable knowledge. The pass rate for this exam has hovered for years in the 50–60 percent range. Of those who pass the writtens, approximately an equal percentage pass the orals. Are those who fail deficient in quality of character, detectable only by oral exam? There is no evidence to support such a view. In fact, statistics suggest that persons who fail the orals the first time can expect to pass if they retake the exam. What is measured, therefore, is endurance, the ability to sustain motivation while waiting to find a set of examiners who will judge an individual's performance to be worthy of certification.

My own experience is consistent with the general pattern. I took my ABPN written exam in the spring of 1974 and passed it. When I took my orals in October of the same year, along with seven hundred other psychiatrists—examining patients in front of examiners who observed and later questioned me about what I had done—I was failed. In addition to being regarded as technically deficient in certain aspects of neurology, I failed the psychiatry portion essentially for what my examiners perceived as aberrations in character. I was seen as "somewhat condescending and nonattentive to the patient as an individual." My examiners thought that I showed "a lack of sensitivity to the patients."

Whatever the merits of these particular observations in the particular circumstances of the examination setting, they were totally at variance with any feedback I have had about my performance at any time in my training or clinical practice. Further, on my next attempt at the orals, only three months after the first, I passed easily, presumably without any significant shifts in my basic character. Instead, I had practiced performing in front of an audience in a series of contrived mock-exams, so that I could present my actual examiners with a reasonably convincing bit of theater.

The purpose of describing this is not to point an accusing finger at persons on examining boards who are struggling to do their best in imperfect circumstances, or to parade my own problems in public, but rather to draw attention to the limitations of mass testing procedures and the kind of game-playing postures that physicians must adopt in order to demonstrate that they can deliver so-called quality care. Any art is ambiguous, but credentials tend not to be. Requirements for technical expertise and standardized behavior will help to mold the kinds of doctors who will care for us in the future.

Among the many aspects of this preoccupation with credentialing that people like Irv and me find particularly galling is the exclusion of the concept of personality "fit" between doctor and patient. Credentialing tends to classify patients by diseases and doctors by technical skills, so that Irv as a psychiatrist might be allowed to care for the "psychiatric" problems of the sergeant and the angry young man he saw in the walk-in clinic, but would not be allowed to care for a pneumonia in either person. That disorder (and the person afflicted with it) would have to be referred to a general practitioner or an internist. Yet Irv, as a physician and psychiatrist, might do better caring for the sergeant's pneumonia than he would treating the young man's impulsive, potentially violent anger. With the sergeant, he has a natural empathy and a comfortable therapeutic relationship, so that the sergeant would tend to trust him, follow his advice, and take the medication Irv prescribed. But if any physician is going to establish such a relationship with the young man in the walk-in clinic, it's clearly not Irv. In taking responsibility for treating both "psychiatric" patients, Irv ends up looking cold and insensitive 50 percent of the time.

There is plenty of room in this world for cold and impersonal physicians. There are certainly plenty of cold and impersonal patients, and numerous medical problems that can usefully be approached in a cold and impersonal fashion. The issue is rather whether the system accepts these differences, and makes allowances for them, so that both doctor and patient are given equal room to be full human beings, or whether the unique personal qualities of the individual physician are gradually being suppressed in the effort to impose homogeneous technical standards.

Continuing medical education is more of the same. Over the past decade, many professional organizations and state licensing boards have begun to require physicians to submit evidence of CME—i.e., of "keeping up with the latest developments." What constitutes acceptable CME? In order to count on a doctor's record, CME must be accredited. Overwhelmingly, CME courses purvey more didactic material: the latest techinques, facts, and numbers.

I don't mean to imply that such courses have no worth; of course they do. I take my share of CME courses, not only because they are required but because I need the instruction to preserve and enhance my skills. What I resent in the process is that the very nature of the courses tends to push medicine further and further toward an overwhelming preoccupation with science and technology, a path that I believe leads to further alienation of doctors and patients without significantly ameliorating the suffering we presume to treat.

There are no CME credits given the pediatrician who becomes the parent of a sick child and learns firsthand what it feels like to sit alongside the bed of one's own ailing infant. The internist gets no CME credit when he or she has a heart attack and suddenly views an intensive care unit from the patient's point of view. No one gives CME credits for spending time with loved ones, or going to church, or struggling with personal priorities and values—even though these activities may make a physician more sensitive and caring. The credentialing pressures point in a different direction.

Another tack in trying to study the quality of care has been to measure so-called process variables. That is, what process does the doctor go through in order to examine and treat the patient and the patient's ills? Though attractive in theory, these measures involve the proliferation of paper. In order to judge a doctor's handiwork, all the appropriate blanks must first be completed in the appropriate manner. In fact, if the chart is filled in correctly, treating the patient becomes a secondary issue, of interest only if obvious discrepancies can be demonstrated between the contents of the chart and the medical course of the patient. Once the blanks are filled in, an auditor clerk can then start collecting statistics to see where an individual physician fits within the broad pattern of the profession. Does this doctor keep patients undergoing appendectomies in the hospital a longer or shorter time than the mode? Does that one order cultures before prescribing antibiotics? Does this physician see as many patients per hour as the others in the clinic, or ask the patients about their sex lives or eating habits?

As I sit in my office in the hospital furiously scribbling down all the details of a patient's condition and planned treatment, patients wander by and wonder what the doctor is doing in there writing when they have been waiting so long to be seen. Their curiosity and irritation are understandable, yet I write at length in the chart not only so that the next doctor who picks it up will understand what has transpired, but because I have to protect myself. I write to demonstrate that I have done a thorough examination, that I have discussed alternatives with the patient, that I have advised and instructed him or her as I should, and that I have arranged sufficient follow-up as needed. Anything less leaves me vulnerable to charges of negligence, to malpractice suits, and to suspicions of incompetence by the quality-assurance monitors. Ironically, it may be more advantageous to me personally to fill in the chart correctly than to treat the patient correctly.

The assumption is that reliance on objective data will allow us to determine who are the good doctors and who are the bad ones, as though the two were clearly separable. We can then suspend or remove the licenses of those whom we label inadequate or incompetent, and pretend that we have remedied one problem without having created another just as grievous.

Not only does the doctor not get points for developing a productive doctor-patient relationship in a system increasingly point-oriented; but spending precious minutes in conversation with patients takes time and emotional energy away from tasks that are both measurable and measured—and for which the doctor will be rewarded by the health-care system.

10 RUSSELL: The Shock Doctor

Visiting Russell at work is like stepping into a prison: the heavy door thuds into the jamb behind me, the key grates metallically in the lock, the tumblers turn noisily, and I am caged inside a ward of the state hospital. I am only a visitor here; I will leave within the hour; but the feeling of confinement is acute. I don't like it at all.

Russell and I are acquaintances and colleagues not friends, though we have known each other in various contexts for years. This time, we have been brought together because we are both members of a committee of our local psychiatric professional organization. We have the task of preparing a program for an upcoming meeting, and we are going at our assignment conscientiously if not enthusiastically. For our previous get-together, working at the same task, we met at a place of my choosing: a little café in the Italian section of San Francisco, a happy place with exuberant frescoes on the walls and ceilings, with delicious cappuccino and pastries, with attractive women and men, people with animated faces and bodies and voices. This time we are meeting at a place of Russell's choosing, one dictated by his cramped schedule.

Russell and I walk down the long corridor toward his office, our footsteps echoing off the state hospital's institutional walls. We pass the nurses' station where patients are lined up to get their medicine. Nearby, an elderly woman is seated in a chrome and green vinyl chair, unkempt head in her hands, sobbing softly. Faces loom at me out of the hallway, and I see them as disconnected from their bodies: vacant eyes, grotesque grins, some of them woeful, some tense, some as ordinary as passengers on a bus.

A pale woman walks up to me as I stride alongside my colleague. "You thought you could burn my city," she says accusingly. "You thought you could get away with it. I'm not going to let you." She's in her fifties, with hair the color of lemon pepper, pulled back untidily in a bun. She wears a tightly buttoned fake leather coat the same color as her hair. Her face is frozen in a toothy grin, eyes the color of wilted lilacs.

I haven't the vaguest notion of what she's talking about, and, in any event, it isn't my responsibility. I'm only a visitor here. I ignore her—and think fleetingly of a line from *The Snake Pit* about psychiatrists "always talking about hearing voices and never hearing mine."

In the distance I can hear a man yelling obscenities, punctuating his words with blows against some solid object. I know what the sounds mean without having to ask: somewhere a patient is locked in a seclusion room, and he wants to be released.

Russell and I settle into his office. Even if I were deaf and blind, I would know what place I was in. It's the smell of institutions, neither dirty nor clean, a blend of human odors and disinfectant. Subtle yet complex, it is the aroma of anonymous history. How many souls have been here, and what tales might they tell if someone had but time to listen? But few people ever do.

I had a moonlighting job for a while at a different state hospital south of San Francisco. I worked at night, as the only physician on duty for twelve hundred hospitalized patients and the only physician available to process the ten to twenty new admissions each night. I carried a master key, which put me in control of the hundreds of locked doors in the place, and a restraint key, which gave me power over the leather restraints with metal locks that some patients wore. As a practical matter, however, I rarely saw any of the hospitalized patients. There simply wasn't time—and even when there was a moment, it was difficult to work up the inclination to carry me from the drab and musty but light and secure administration building, out into the dark and ghostly grounds, and from there into the frightening wards housing the frightened and sometimes frightening people who fill such places. If I saw one patient on a ward, I would have been exposed to the unanswerable demands of hundreds; and the prospect was too intimidating. Instead, I stayed in my little office, processing the new admissions and dealing with problems over the phone: ordering sedation for patient after patient after patient, relying on the nurses' discretion and experience for drug and dosage choice. I dealt with people on paper and people en masse, and tried to convince myself that despite my behavior I was a good physician. In the year I worked there, I developed a profound respect for doctors, nurses, and others who could work in such places and somehow retain their humanity and dedication to patient care.

Russell's office is in a smallish room whose two windows are barred to discourage persons thinking of using them for an unauthorized exit. In an effort to cheer the place up, someone decided to accent the hospital walls with wide stripes in primary colors. The stripe on two of the walls in Russell's office is a bold yellow.

"What's the story of the shouter?" I ask.

Russell replies: "He was brought in by the police. He'd been downtown, going up to women on the street, yelling at them, calling them sluts and seductresses. If he had been a smaller or older man, the officers probably would have just told him to move along and left it at that. But he's big and rather terrifying to look at, and he weighs over two hundred and twenty pounds, so the police officers decided to take him in for safety's sake. Since he is clearly psychotic, talking about being the vengeful angel of God, they brought him here instead of to jail."

"What do you do with a guy like that?"

"What do you think?" he asks me rhetorically, his tone implying that I'm a ninny. "We can't let him wander around the ward because he'll terrorize the women and get into fights with the men. So we put him in seclusion and we medicate him. If we don't medicate him, he'll keep everybody awake at night and put everybody's nerves on edge all day with his yelling. This place is tense enough without that kind of aggravation. Every time we open the door to the seclusion room to feed him or do a physical exam on him, he'll slug one of the attendants. So we give him a healthy dose of medication; and if that doesn't work, we give him more medication until it does work.

There's nothing else you can do. The problem, of course, is that he won't take the medication voluntarily, so we have to get a bunch of burly attendants in here to strap him down so we can give him the medication by injection."

Russell looks at me. My discomfort with what he says must show, or perhaps his own uneasiness prompts him. Russell has gotten very sensitive to criticism about brutality toward patients since he was listed by one of the antipsychiatry groups in something called the "Shock Doctor Register," a nationally distributed roster of psychiatrists who administer electroshock therapy (abbreviated ECT, for electroconvulsive therapy). In the aftermath, Russell has received numerous poisonous letters and phone calls implying that he is cruel and insensitive, a Gestapo guard masquerading as a doctor.

"Look," he continues, "if you think we enjoy this kind of confrontation, you're mistaken. We like to see ourselves as healers and helpers, not jailers and goons. The last time our attendants had to tackle a fellow this big, one of them got a nasty bite, another got a bloody nose, and a third got kneed in the groin. There's no satisfaction in this kind of endeavor at all, and there's a lot of aggravation. It's just part of the job, that's all."

Russell continues to peer at me, watching for a reaction. Why do I feel so uncomfortable?

"Without chemical treatment, we wouldn't have a chance at the talking cure," he goes on. "How can you carry on a conversation with one patient when a dozen others are screaming and throwing tantrums? You can't do it."

On the wall above the desk are his diplomas and certificates: medical school, internship, residency, specialty board, medical licensure—credentials which document that Russell is an heir to the Hippocratic tradition. The ornaments of a professional life. He's a physician, like me, dedicated to healing the sick. On either side are some Audubon prints of ornately colored birds, gorgeous creatures, each depicted in airy flight. On the desk is an expensive pair of binoculars. Russell is a bird-watcher, and sometimes he manages to catch a glimpse of a rare specimen in the field beyond his office window. The hospital sits in the path of the migratory species who use the Pacific Flyway. Outside the window, a misty rain is falling, soundless, gray, and drab.

"How many of your patients are like the shouter?" I ask.

"It depends what you mean. He's bigger and louder and more violent than most, but he's typical in that none of the patients would choose to be here if they had anyplace else to go. No one goes to the state hospital who doesn't have to. You've got to be crazy, either literally or figuratively, to be a patient here. Most patients resent being here and resent the staff. They want to get out of here, but they see their need for change as something that is being externally imposed. Helping them is like trying to help a wild alley cat with a thorn in its paw. What the staff wants to do is remove the thorn, but in order to do that you have to first win the cat's trust—which may take forever, if it's possible at all—or you have to overpower the poor unfortunate creature, making sure all the time that you don't get scratched or bitten, and that the cat's yowling or spitting doesn't deter you from your task."

"So much for the doctor-patient, relationship," I say, my tone of voice harsher than I had intended.

"Are you kidding?" Russell is incredulous that I even say such a thing. "Our census runs about forty patients per day on this ward, but with turnover we probably see about sixty individual patients here each week. If I spend forty hours a week just seeing patients, individually at an hour a crack, I'd see each patient every one and a half weeks. That's not counting administrative stuff, court appearances, meeting with staff, meeting with families, writing orders in the chart, writing reports, or time out for going to the bathroom. As a practical matter, I probably only spend ten hours a week in direct patient contact, which averages out to about ten minutes per patient per week. How can you form a doctor-patient relationship under circumstances like that? Almost all the patients here have to be taken care of by other staff nominally under my supervision.

"You've got to understand what it's like here. We have a constant influx of patients and a finite number of places to put them. That means we have to constantly be discharging patients. It doesn't matter whether they're better than when they came in. We hope they are. We hope the ones going out are in better shape than the ones coming in—but it doesn't really matter. Unless people are totally unable to function, the law won't allow us to keep them—and we haven't got the space to keep them anyway. What they do between the time they come in and the time they leave we call treatment. The welfare of the patient is incidental, and professional judgment is almost irrelevant. The patients' legal condition is more important than their clinical condition."

It's not by accident that Russell's special professional interest is masochism. He's written several papers on the topic for professional journals. Actually, it's the story of his life: the pursuit of virtue through suffering. He believes that doing a hard job well is a measure of character, and that's what life for a responsible person is all about. His father was a preacher, a stern man with little tolerance for jokes or horseplay. Russell was a serious, responsible youngster, and he has become a serious, responsible adult, reserved with strangers, almost shy. There's a countrified dignity to him, a loquacious somber pessimism. He doesn't simply talk, he lectures. It's not hard to imagine him as a preacher whose view of life is dominated by the book of Job.

The door opens suddenly, and a scarecrow of a man walks in. He's wearing old black tennis shoes and a faded, dirty brown-and-white jogging suit. His gaunt face a mass of lines, it looks ravaged by a half century of agony. But he moves with the agility of a much younger man, and I estimate that he is about thirty. His eyes are wide with fear, and he says to Russell: "The spirits are telling me evil things again. They are making me think bad thoughts." His voice is dry and rasping, and it has a hat-in-hand pleading quality.

Russell responds: "Go tell the nurse and he'll give you some medicine"—but the man stands rooted to the spot, staring at Russell.

"All right," Russell says with a sigh. He gets up and takes the man by the elbow and leads him from my line of vision. When Russell returns, he sits in his chair once more and says: "The staff was in a meeting."

I nod my head. Meetings aren't just for transacting institutional business. The staff in mental institutions tends to spend a lot of time in meetings. Ostensibly meetings are held for the communication of information and judgments about the patients and patient care. Seminars, conferences, reports (they are called a variety of names) also provide an opportunity for the staff to cling to one another—the presumably sane—for support and reassurance and guidance. It's too risky being with those patients all the time. Their despair and anguish and craziness are contagious. The staff needs a break from it all. Even so, individuals who work in mental hospitals for very long tend to develop little quirks, little peculiarities, little neurotic patterns. I don't like to think what would happen to my personality and well-being if I worked in such a place.

"Let's get to work," I say, and we spend the next thirty minutes hammering out details of the program that is our assignment: the speaker, who will introduce him, the discussants, ticket prices, refreshments, publicity—all the petty things that remain of trivial importance only so long as they go smoothly.

The joint effort creates a bond between us where before there was awkward tension, and Russell relaxes and warms up a bit, and I guess I do too. He asks me how I have been doing since my divorce, and I tell him. He asks me how my parents are doing, and I tell him that too. He knows about my mother's cancer of the esophagus and her difficult operation and postoperative course. He knows about my father's multiple sclerosis, and his increasing disability and invalidism over the past twenty-five years. He asks about my well-being with practiced skill. Inquiring after people's welfare is a professional occupation for both of us, but our empathy with each other is genuine enough.

Russell's adolescence was even more influenced by sickness than was mine. His grade-school and high-school years in Kentucky were dominated by the illness of his sister, two years his senior. She developed a rare neurological disease and gradually lost all power in her limbs. Slowly the deterioration spread to her speech, her intellect, her bowel and bladder. Russell's mother nursed her during the day to the point of exhaustion; and after school, in the evenings, and on weekends and vacations, it was Russell's duty to spell her. It was more than that too: it was an opportunity for giving and a labor of love— but at a cost. His was not a happy home, and he was not a happy child.

"How are you doing since your wife's death?" I ask him. His wife died in an automobile accident seven months ago. She was driving alone on a clear night, and went off a cliff on the coastal highway. Rumor has it that she was drunk and had been taking a lot of pills. I don't know for sure, and I haven't asked Russell directly. Some people have speculated that her accident was essentially a suicidal act. I don't know the truth of that either, but what a bitter irony if it's true: a psychiatrist's spouse committing suicide.

"I'm coping," he says. "I'm trying to spend more time with the kids. It's been hardest on them. But they seem to be adjusting."

Russell has four children, the oldest seventeen and the youngest six. He has never felt he had enough time and emotional energy to give all that was asked of him at home and at the hospital. He relied heavily on his wife to look after things at home, and she felt she had to be both father and mother.

When he came home at the end of a workday, after being surround-ed by agony and people struggling often vainly to be helped and to be of help, the last thing he wanted to hear were his family's problems. He had little tolerance for listening to his kids talk about school trou-bles or his wife talk about car troubles—or neighbor troubles or trou-bles with relatives. What he wanted was peace and quiet. Some soli-tude. Some nurturing. Maybe an undisturbed hour pruning silent fruit trees in his backyard. Maybe some unmeasured minutes watch-ing and listening to the birds of the dusk, who sing their cheery songs and expect nothing of him in return.

His wife resented his lack of givingness at home. He knew that his family deserved more, but he never felt that he had more in him. The patient comes first, he always believed and always said, and the pa-tient is getting short shrift as it is.

Once, shortly before she was killed, I saw Russell's wife at a party. She had had a good bit to drink. The subject of a physician's emo-tional overinvolvement in work came up—the "I-gave-at-the-office" syndrome—and it prompted her to tell a story. It seemed that every-one in her six-year-old son's first-grade class had been asked what they wanted to be when they grew up. When her son's turn came, he said: "*I* want to be a patient."

"Isn't that a scream?" Russell's wife had said. "Isn't that a god-damn scream?"—and she laughed so bitterly that people edged away from her.

Her palpable resentment had prompted a discussion among several of us about how sagging morale among many clinicians was related to the decline and fall of the doctor's wife as a respected social institu-tion. How can physicians be expected to provide a reliable source of solace to others when there is no stable support system in the back-ground? When even the idea of a traditionally devoted spouse, who has given up a separate career in order to be supportive to a mate, is increasingly subject to ridicule? Like most such cocktail party chat-ter, the conversation got nowhere—and after a while we shifted to less uncomfortable topics.

"How are you doing at being both a mother and a father?" I now asked Russell.

"My seventeen-year-old takes a fair amount of responsibility for running the home," he responds, "and the fifteen-year-old and ten-year-old are pretty good too. I hired a housekeeper who looks after things on weekdays, and I try to spend all my weekends with the kids.

We're getting along." He pauses, and then adds: "In many ways, my three oldest kids are more understanding of my work commitment than my wife was. They all want to be lawyers, and I'm encouraging them."

"Why is that?" I ask. I know that Russell blames the legal profession for many of the hassles of his working day.

"Because law is in ascendancy," he says. "Most of the therapeutic decisions and interventions of the future will be made in a legal arena. Practically everything we do here now is subject to external scrutiny and regulation. It's like working in a glass cage where you've got to follow somebody else's rules, but the rules and the people making them keep changing.

"All this recent litigation and legislation has developed new standards for rights to receive treatment, rights to refuse treatment, rights of confidentiality, and rights to have customary confidentiality disregarded. There is a movement to require judicial and/or committee approval for a variety of treatment decisions, even for such traditional medical judgments as giving a common injectable medication without the patient's explicit consent, or raising the dosage of some common tranquilizers above arbitrarily established levels. I heard that in Massachusetts fifteen hospitalized patients sued their doctors in a hospital because they felt they were being overmedicated. The American Civil Liberties Union has instituted a suit designed to require judicial review before medications can be raised above certain arbitrary levels. The effect is to make it a right for patients to have judicial review before receiving many medications at effective dose levels. If the suit is decided solely on judicial grounds, and not on medical or practical grounds, it will probably be decided in favor of mandatory review. In the future, every time we order a medication, the dosage will be a matter to be decided before a court of law. The effect will be to take clinical judgment away from the physician and give it to the judge. Perhaps the judges will do a better job than the doctors, and perhaps not—but it is clear that they are going to have increasing responsibility for such decisions."

Soon they are going to have to start selling judges malpractice insurance, I think to myself. I'm only half listening to Russell. All the rules and regulations give me a pain. Who can keep track of them? Who wants to? If I were interested in this kind of thing, I would have gone to law school or married a lawyer. I nod to Russell to indicate I'm still following him. I know that the point he is trying to make is an important one. Despite my flip internal responses, I know I can't avoid the issue any more easily than he can.

He continues, his voice even. "What that means is that I'll have to go to court to request an adequate dosage, and I'll be represented by a lawyer, and the patient will be there too, also represented by a lawyer—and the arguments will be about motives and character, whether or not I'm cruel or malicious or sadistic, and not about dose-effectiveness curves and psychopharmacology, which none of the laymen will be equipped to understand anyhow. The immediate effect of all this will be to keep drug levels lower, so as to avoid all legalistic hassles. I can't be going to court over dosage decisions all the time; I'm not spending enough time with patients as it is. So most physicians will lean toward undertreatment rather than overtreatment.

"That in itself might not be so bad, but they've got us there too. The Donaldson decision maintains that every hospitalized patient has the right to adequate treatment, and if we undertreat the patients, treat them inadequately, then we'll be legally liable for the failure to achieve positive results.

"I think the long-term effect of all this will simply be to drive conscientious clinicians from the care of the sickest patients. No matter what the situation, there is potential legal liability for action and an equally ominous liability for inaction. Either they get you for what they call negligence or for what they call assault. I'm telling you—the future lies with the lawyers."

I look at my companion, his thin blond hair like cornsilk, precisely trimmed, sideburns shaved high, wearing a suit jacket and tie despite the sweat collecting on his brow in the high humidity. He is wearing a lime-green shirt and an off-yellow tie. The colors are all wrong for him, giving his face an unhealthy pallor.

He has a thin, sardonic smile on his face, but beneath the superficial certainty lies gloomy resignation. I can smell depression in the room, and it's not all mine. Russell thinks he has identified the opposition—the lawyers—and since he can't beat them, he plans to join them, using his children as emissaries to the enemy camp. His own frustration and feelings of inadequacy become tolerable and even tinged with hope, now that he has identified what he perceives as the powerful elite of the future.

I sit silently, moodily. I don't like approaching problem-solving by calling some people enemies. I doubt that the legal profession will have any more success in dealing with craziness than has psychiatry. I know a lot of lawyers, and they're struggling too. Those of them who work in the mental-health arena are in as much of a muddle as the psychiatrists.

"Here's a perfect example," he continues. "I have a lady on the ward now who wants to kill herself. Everybody agrees to that, including her. She wants to leave and jump off the bridge, so we are keeping her here against her will—in part because that's what the law requires and in part because her family says they will sue me if she commits suicide. But I can't treat her. Medications don't help her at all, and I'm not allowed to give ECT, which I think is the treatment of choice. The law says that I can't give her ECT against her will; if I do, I am liable to a fine of five thousand dollars and suspension of my license. The irony is that she was hospitalized for exactly the same problem five years ago, got a short course of ECT over her protests, and got along wonderfully up to last month."

Russell is suddenly quiet, and as I look at him the signs of weariness fairly jump out at me: the stooped shoulders, the pinched mouth, the melancholy eyes peeking out from beneath dark and puffy lids. I know that morale is terrible amongst psychiatrists at the state hospital. Many who have had other places to go have simply quit. They can't take it very long. They all burn out. The ones who don't leave end up developing an emotional suit of armor so thick that they don't feel anything with their patients.

I shift uncomfortably in my chair. I want to get up and get out and leave this place. Russell and his staff are performing a public service. My training has equipped me to perform likewise, and yet I have no taste for it. I respect him for doing what I cannot, especially now with the pain of his wife's death so fresh in his experience.

"What keeps you here, Russell?" I ask. "Why do you stay?"

"What's a person to do, Marty? There's so much pain out there. If someone like me won't help people with it, who will? I look at my burned-out co-workers and wonder if I'll end up like them. Sometimes I think the key to emotional survival is just not thinking about things too much, not feeling too much. But if I do that, what kind of therapist, what kind of person would I be? Sometimes I think the bureaucratic structure and my role in it serve to protect me from the contagious craziness of the patients. But the more bureaucratic the structure, the less we get back as human beings too. I don't want to wall off my feelings, but I'm afraid not to."

He looks at me intently for a moment and says, "There's a line from *The Myth of Sisyphus* by Camus. Maybe you know it. 'The gods had condemned Sisyphus to ceaselessly rolling a rock to the top of a mountain, whence the stone would fall back of its own weight. They had thought with some reason that there is no more dreadful punishment than futile and hopeless labor.' "

What is there I can possibly say? Russell is trapped by his own dedication and commitment in an institutional framework where each new calendar leaf is filled primarily by frustration. He calls an attendant to show me to the door, shakes my hand, and waves a distracted good-bye.

As I step outside the ward, the door once again thuds behind me, this time with me on the outside, as the key tumbles the lock closed. The rain has stopped and the sky is surprisingly bright, with a few tardy clouds not yet pushed eastward by the strong wind that is blowing. The blue jays are out in force on the hospital grounds, raucous, mocking, and free.

I'm relieved to be out of confinement, out in the sunshine, smelling the eucalyptus trees as I walk to my car. What was it Russell had said? The effect of all the litigation will be to drive clinicians from the care of the sickest patients.

Driving home, I ponder my collegial responsibility to Russell, sitting in his cage of an office. I think the man is barely holding on. What are my obligations to him? It's a professional as well as a personal question.

And yet it is not. In Russell's world and increasingly in mine, professional responsibility is well-defined. A physician has responsibility only to his assigned patients or to patients with whom he has some sort of contractual arrangement enforceable by law. Our professions's traditional obligation to assist anyone in need is now clearly an idealistic fantasy, if in fact it ever was more than that. There are simply too many people in need. No individual can assume responsibility for helping everyone in pain whom he or she encounters along the road. I doubt that any single profession can assume such a burden.

To hell with it, I tell myself. It's Russell's life. He's an adult. He's as responsible a person as anyone I know, more so than most. Who am I to intrude?

I grip the wheel and drive very carefully. The fragility of life and sanity requires a tight grip on the wheel, and I can drive only one car at a time.

11 THE DOCTOR-PATIENT RELATIONSHIP: Assembly-Line Medicine

At the time I saw Russell, I was chairman of the Well-Being Committee of my local psychiatric professional organization. That meant I was the person who would be called if someone felt that a psychiatrist in our geographical area was struggling or in need of some collegial help. As such, you would think I'd know what to do if I were concerned about someone like Russell. Our committee, after all, had spent the better part of the year developing a protocol to guide our actions when we received word of a colleague who was floundering.

But though the steps outlined in the protocol made sense when I was counseling a stranger, it seemed to me too mechanical an approach with someone I knew. In a bizarre way, the idea of invoking the protocol with Russell—utilizing an institutional response in an intensely personal situation—typified the very set of circumstances that ensnared Russell. Russell is himself a product of institutionalized therapeutics.

Whatever his strengths and weaknesses—and, like all of us, he has his share of both—Russell strives to be a decent person, to conduct his professional activities with integrity and sensitivity, yet he is not being very successful at adapting his personal qualities to the institutional setting in which he practices his profession. His innate gentleness, thoughtfulness, and compassion are qualities that probably few of his patients perceive. These qualities seem totally absent from his ward milieu. Even worse, he feels his capacity for caring being overwhelmed, and he senses that deep within him he is becoming crass, brutal, and coarse.

We know that institutions have the power to mold character, in adults as well as children; but we have not yet come to terms with the influence of modern industrialized medicine on the practitioners who labor within its boundaries.

Try to imagine an old village blacksmith—a person most of us know from fiction or verse if at all—laboring within a General Motors assembly plant. The blacksmith's essential qualities—the ability to individually craft a shoe to a particular horse, the temperament to work alone for long hours in a pastoral stable full of four-legged creatures, the patience and sensitivity to gain the confidence of spirited and often frightened animals—these qualities not only have little use on an assembly line, but they are counterproductive. A good blacksmith would be a poor assembly-line worker.

Yet we are training all our doctors to be assembly-line workers, and more and more we view medical care as a commodity to be judged by assembly-line standards.

Without taking away one whit from the discomfort of patients in depersonalized health-care institutions, it's useful to understand that the situation is equally impersonal from the viewpoint of most students and staff. The system is set up to function regardless of who occupies a given bed at a given moment—or who is treating the patient at that moment. The identity of a patient in a given bed may change every few days and the identity of a given student or house officer may change every few weeks, but from the point of view of the system, each group is equally faceless. The pattern is most dramatically clear in training institutions where the turnover in staff is unending; but it is also obvious in group practices where unfamiliar physicians take call for familiar ones—and where the on-call physician sees patients who are largely strangers to him or her.

When patients see me in the emergency room or drop-in clinic, they do so not because they are attracted to me personally or because they value my skill or reputation, but because I am *there* and they need a service provided by an accessible someone with suitable credentials. Once they see me, if I should decide they need additional services, perhaps for a dermatologic or surgical problem that is beyond my skill to diagnose or treat, I refer them to the dermatology clinic or the surgery clinic. The specific doctor who will see a patient is usually irrelevant; the job will be performed by a suitably credentialed body in an institutional slot.

This process does not occur only in metropolitan medical practice. The equivalent goes on in smaller towns everywhere. Even a little place like Alturas, California, population 3,000, flies in rent-a-docs, strangers from out of town, to provide needed services on a rotating basis. It's part of a nationwide system. More and more health care is being given by institutions, not by individuals. More and more care is being dispensed in emergency rooms, where the identity of the physician on duty at a specific time is often totally unpredictable from the patient's point of view. Though many adults will have had experience with personal physicians in the past, a growing number of young people have never had a doctor of their own and presumably never expect to. They are the impersonal recipients of the impersonal care of the future.

Impersonality is not simply an unavoidable side effect; it is an integral in the design of the system. As in any good production unit, not only must the parts that constitute the work of the assembly line be interchangeable, but the workers themselves must be interchangeable.

Both the patient and the people caring for the patient must behave in a standardized, replicable manner in order for the system to function efficiently. There is not only little time for idiosyncrasy; there is no room for rapport. There is certainly no time for the assembly-line worker to gaze fondly, thoughtfully, at his contribution to the final product. The line must keep moving.

Doctors who resist the process inevitably become subjected to bureaucratic pressures. If their "stats"—the number of patients seen per unit of time—don't match the institutional norm, they must either shape up and speed up, or find another job.

Patients who resist processing and who slow up the production line—those who demand to be treated as full human beings or who don't present their problems concisely and in a manner that makes them readily soluble—are regarded as difficult patients, troublemakers, and they soon collect a variety of derogatory labels: "hypochondriac," "manipulator," "personality disorder."

It's not that we doctors lack humanity per se. Rather, we have come to understand what most patients as yet do not: we must find ways of distancing ourselves from them, and limiting our emotional responsibility to them, when the dimensions of their problems overwhelm not only our therapeutic skills but our constricted and enfeebled role on the production line.

Health care is an industry; and the training which individuals get in order to participate in that industry presupposes that diseases constitute essentially replicable items, that the skills necessary to treat diseases are definable in technical terms and replicable, and that the consequences of treatment are both measurable and subject to cost-effectiveness analysis.

In order for physician behavior to be consistent with the biomedical technological model, that behavior must also be definable, measurable, and codifiable. Any behavior that is not codifiable has no value and must be discouraged as taking up time which could be devoted to codifiable behavior. Most codifiable behaviors are subject to considerable scrutiny with regard to a dominant criterion: does each behavior help the health-care production lines flow more smoothly or not? If not, how can the organization of the production line be changed to facilitate greater efficiency? Individual misery and attempts to alleviate it must be reducible to administrative terms.

Russell sits at one spot on one of the specialized production lines. He sees only the regulations, feels only his own impotence and impersonality, and finds it difficult to gain a perspective that allows him to feel he matters. He is dimly aware that he has become a cog in an immense and incomprehensible machine, and he doesn't like it. When he thinks about it, he tends to blame his troubles on people belonging to the antipsychiatry movement and their legal advisors—and he complains a lot, which sometimes makes it tedious to listen to him.

I see the phenomenon as far broader than that. The production-line mentality has Russell sharing a common plight with obstetricians in a local obstetrics and gynecology clinic. They schedule one woman patient every seven and a half minutes. The doctor comes into the examining room where the patient is already up in stirrups, feels the abdomen, does the pelvic examination, orders laboratory tests, writes a prescription, and is gone. There is no time for any discussion, no time for rapport, no time to assess the patient's understanding of the examination or treatment. The production-line concept of medical care forbids it.

Whenever I say this to lay people, the first response is always: "Well if doctors weren't so money-grubbing, they would take more time with patients."

Although that observation may sometimes be true, it is not the most important factor in this particular circumstance. These obstetricians are all salaried. They get no more money for seeing more patients. Most of them are in specialty training, essentially transients in the clinic, and they have little opportunity to influence clinic policy. The clinic makes more money by seeing more patients, but the clinic is state-owned, a unit in a so-called nonprofit institution, and the institution is chronically in the red anyhow. Physicians' salaries account for only a small percentage of the outlays from patient fees. Money is a relevant concern, but only one of many. Among others, the rapid rate at which patient appointments are scheduled is a response to the continuing press of patients. The waiting room is always full. The appointment list is booked for weeks in advance. San Francisco has one of the highest doctor-patient ratios in the country, yet the press of patients awaiting appointments never abates.

The obstetricians in this example are required, by the nature of the organization of their work, to focus their attention on one aspect of the patients' bodies. They simply haven't time for anything more— for talking about feelings or anxieties, or for treating the patient's cold or ingrown toenail for that matter. If one obstetrician insists on taking extra time, that doctor's patients will have to wait even longer than they do already, or that doctor's colleagues will have to work even faster to compensate for one of their number going more slowly.

Most people don't like the cool impersonality of the seven-and-a-half-minute obstetrician. They ask: "What's wrong with doctors? I want a doctor to treat me like a human being, not as just another pelvis hanging from a pair of stirrups."

Of course people want to be treated like human beings. Of course. Unfortunately, people also want a lot of other things which will make that kind of treatment less and less likely in the future. For instance, they want technical excellence. Though the narrow focus of the seven-and-a-half-minute obstetrician prohibits a more comprehensive approach to the patient, those doctors who perform eight pelvic exams in an hour and thirty pelvic exams in an afternoon tend to become very, very competent at their narrowly defined, highly specialized task. This level of competence among trainees at a prestigious medical center sets standards in turn for the rest of us physicians. From a systems analyst's point of view, these obstetricians are superb and efficient technicians: they do a high volume of procedures (each pelvic exam is one procedure), attain considerable hard data (each Pap smear, culture, or other laboratory test result is quantifiable information), and uncover a significant amount of codifiable disease. The average generalist judged by the same standards would be found wanting. In caring for the whole patient—or in attempting to do so—no one aspect of that care can match a specialist's intensity, brisk efficiency, or level of achievement.

One would think that there would be room in professional standards for variations due to locale, breadth of clinical focus, personal style, and so forth—but in practice the trend is in the opposite direction. Just because I—or any other physician—try to take care of a patient as a whole human being does not mean that I should be allowed substantially more time than the specialist for doing a pelvic exam, or that I should be given special dispensation if I fail to diagnose a tumor in the uterus that a specialist might more likely have uncovered. The tendency is to apply a specialist's standards both in terms of economy of time and in terms of results—not only in malpractice cases, but also in the criteria physicians apply to their own performance. If a woman succumbs to cancer of the uterus because she was examined by me instead of a gynecologist, how can I conscientiously continue to practice with the superficial knowledge of a generalist as opposed to the more profound accomplishment of a specialist?

Generalists are not only becoming more improbable, but they will soon be illegal. Not in name, of course. Everyone will continue to pay lip service to the importance of generalists, and everyone will bemoan the lack of good ones. But for all practical purposes, generalists will be regulated and sued and credentialed and demoralized out of business. The general practitioner will be afraid to treat a sore throat or do a rectal exam without calling in a consultant, lest he be made out to be an incompetent by a malpractice lawyer who will contend that a specialist could have done the job better.

In production-line medicine, legal wariness also affects not only individuality but physicians' willingness to confront difficult clinical challenges. They face not only a lack of reward, but also the very real threat of punishment. Every time I see a potentially suicidal patient who doesn't want to be hospitalized, or a contentious drunk in the emergency room with a head laceration and possible concussion, I wonder: Is this someone who will sue if I treat involuntarily, or am I more likely to be sued for negligence if I don't treat and the patient suffers as a consequence? My stomach lining gnaws at me when I worry defensively about such self-protective questions, but I know that many physicians share my concerns.

Too often we have become mere bystanders to our patients' misery, not because we are crass or because our tools are limited but because treatment decisions are no longer matters to be decided solely by physicians, and doctors increasingly sense that their hands are tied; they feel unable to respond creatively to individual patients' problems. Russell's being barred from treating a seriously depressed patient with the ECT that had previously been life-saving is only one example, but one symptomatic of a trend.

Many institutions that provide patient care now have protocols that dictate the sequence of responses for common health-care problems. For instance, if a patient comes in with a sore throat, the doctor should do this and this; and if the laboratory test produces a certain result, the doctor should also do that and that. Generally these protocols are justified—as most policy decisions in the health arena are justified—in the name of improving patient care. A secondary consideration has to do with efficient use of resources: if the doctor is told precisely what to do, no "unnecessary" tests and medications will be ordered. A third and more cynical view of protocols in this age of monstrous malpractice suits is that they constitute a means for the institutions to cover their collective asses and call the process science.

None of these conceptualizations recognizes that only the exercise of discretion allows for the individualization of the patient and the doctor and the relationship between them. Furthermore, where a course of action is unclear, where the patient's clinical condition requires the doctor to struggle with diagnostic or therapeutic ambiguities, there is less and less incentive for the doctor to use that discretion. The present processes of training discourage it, and the political realities of contemporary practice discourage it. It's always safer to call in consultants or buck difficult decisions to a committee, not because the results for the patient will be any better—or certainly any cheaper—but because responsibility will be diffused.

We are condemned to another paradox: the more conscientiously we try to live by uniform professional standards, the less individuality we feel and the less we can individualize our care of patients. Patients who demand that we treat them as individuals simply confront us with a discrepancy between our historic ideals and the realities of assembly-line medicine. Within that confrontation, we feel frustrated and inept—and often resentful of the person or persons who bring these feelings to our awareness.

God help us, we begin to resent our patients.

12 WARREN: Doctor or Double Agent

Warren is Ferdinand the Bull in pink and grays. He is a big man, well over six feet, with lots of flesh on his body, and craggy features. The effect is dramatized by a bristling seafoam beard and a luxuriant mane of silver hair.

Despite his formidable appearance, Warren is scared: scared for his life and for that of his wife and children. He's scared of his patients, and with good reason.

Warren walked a meandering path before he found himself in psychiatry. He was a high-school dropout, a tempestuous adolescent, given to proud brawling over what he regarded as matters of principle. He fled from home at age seventeen and took up a series of jobs conspicuous for the male camaraderie they provided. He worked heavy construction as a laborer in the Midwest, spent time in a logging camp in Washington state, hired on as a deckhand on a crabbing boat out of the Aleutian Islands, and did a stint as a bartender in a sailors' bar in San Diego. On his twenty-fourth birthday, he and a male friend were out celebrating with two girls they had only recently met. They were all drinking straight whiskey, and no one had sense enough to stay out of the car. None of the survivors even remembered the accident; they were all too drunk. The boy driving came out with minor injuries, but the girl next to him was dead. Warren had compound fractures of both thighs, and his female companion suffered multiple injuries from which she eventually recovered.

During the three months that Warren was in traction on the orthopedic ward, a crucial evolution occurred in his own consciousness. His turbulent, purposeless existence troubled him deeply, and he resolved to find a sense of direction for his own life. The days of enforced inactivity were an unaccustomed agony for him, but they led to a wonderful insight: he enjoyed being reflective, delighted in touring the fascinating recesses of his own mind. He also came to respect the process of caring for sick people and envied the satisfaction the doctors seemed to get from their work. After three months of hospitalization, he decided he wanted to be a physician.

It wasn't easy for him. He had to go back to high school and then put in a stunning performance at junior college so he could get into the university and then into medical school. All the while, he held down a job, sometimes several, on the side. His family had no money, and he wouldn't have asked them for help anyway. He was too independent. Throughout medical school Warren was a loner, set apart from his fellow students by his greater age and the studied snobbism of an intellectual, working-class chauvinist. Warren liked men and women with calluses on their hands and adventurous but thoughtful words on their tongues. He felt ill at ease among his largely middle-class schoolmates and sought out friendships in working-class bars where his county hospital patients hung out.

Warren's father was a cabinetmaker, a fine craftsman when he wasn't drinking, a man of passion and dogma. Warren's mother worked wherever there was a job, and sought solace in her Bible and the book club discussions at her church. Like her husband, she was spirited and opinionated; but her opinions were often at variance with those of her spouse, and the two were recurrently at war. As difficult as they were to live with, Warren loved them from a distance and increasingly appreciated their vibrance and lack of sham.

At the end of medical school, Warren decided, somewhat to his own surprise, that he wanted to go into psychiatry. He understood the choice poorly at the time and feels relatively clear about it only in retrospect.

"I was suspicious of psychiatry's cant and rhetoric and theorizing," he says, "but it seemed to me to offer the greatest job opportunity in the world: a vehicle for spending a lifetime trying to understand human minds and actions. That was the conscious part of my specialty choice. The other part was a poorly distilled desire to come to terms with some of the psychological issues still unresolved from my hellion days, and I think I wanted to find some way to patch up my tattered relationship with my parents."

Now, twenty years later, Warren works in a community mental health center (CMHC) which serves a predominantly blue-collar and unemployed population. He still enjoys seeking to understand troubled minds and feels gratified when he can be helpful. He would never be cruel or insensitive to someone who was suffering or vulnerable; but he increasingly believes that many people who are called patients are neither suffering nor vulnerable, but come to see him for some other reason. Either they are forced to see him by some third party, most commonly the courts, or they come because they want something.

Warren and I used to meet for a few beers after work every now and then at one of the bars near his CMHC. They were all seedy-looking places, inhospitable to an outsider, but with a gruff acceptance and intimacy once you were regarded as a regular. Our favorite was a block away from the CMHC. With a weathered brick exterior and small, high windows, partially screened by neon beer signs, it wasn't much to look at on the outside. The usual claque of winos standing in front, barely able to stand, pulling long gulps surreptitiously from paper-bag clad bottles, hardly seemed much of an endorsement. Inside, there was a marvelous old mahogany bar which had been brought to San Francisco around the Horn in a clipper ship. Everything had a comfortable worn feeling to it. The wooden barstools had been burnished by thousands of rear ends. The mottled beveled mirrors in the ornately carved back bar always held room for another face. Dented spittoons at either end of the bar somehow never got removed, despite repeated warnings from the health department. The patrons were Warren's kind of people: men from a nearby lumber yard, a few ironworkers, an industrial refrigeration salesman, old merchant sailors who had gravitated to shore jobs at the corner ship chandlery, workingman poets—persons of toil and prejudice, broad experience and unadvertised wisdom.

Warren was a great favorite in the bar. He spun out intricate stories with roguish endings. He ranted and stormed in political discussions. He knew all the statistics and all the scores in all the muscular games, yet he didn't hide the soft, sentimental side of his character either. He was a sucker for a sad story, and he willingly emptied out his wallet to a stranger with a sad though improbable tale. That bar seemed to bring out the sweetness and grace in him. He bearhugged men friends just as he did women friends, and kissed them noisily with a booming, "Goddamn, I like you!"

We don't go to that bar any more. Once Warren started becoming afraid, when he began to take the threats seriously, we switched to a bar across town where no one knows him.

"Everywhere I drive," he says, "I'm always looking in the rearview mirror. I don't even know what the hell I'm looking for. Before I park the car, I drive around the block to look for anything suspicious, and in the neighborhood where I work there are always suspicious people. I try to vary my routine every day, but the irony is that in some ways I feel more secure with routine than with doing new things. Every time I see a new patient or somebody I don't know well, I worry that this is the son of a bitch who wants to kill me. I'm wary with practically everyone. This fear is playing havoc with my relationships with patients."

Warren now carries an automatic pistol with him wherever he goes. So does his wife. Both they and their two teenage daughters went to a firing range daily for almost a month to learn to use handguns. Warren's wife drives the daughters everywhere. He worries most about his daughters. "Thank God they haven't started dating yet; I don't know how we could protect them then. I hate to think what this is doing to them. Jesus, God, I hate to think of them growing up scared."

The first note came a year ago, addressed to him at his CMHC office, and said "SUPERSHRINK YOU THINK YOU ARE SO SMART I'M GOING TO GET YOU." They've come at irregular intervals since then, sometimes making obscene comments about his wife and daughters, and always threatening.

Warren thinks he knows who is responsible for the notes, but can't prove it, is not even sure he's right. Two and a half years ago, he participated in a murder trial, testifying grudgingly as an expert witness concerning the sanity of the defendant. Warren hates being in the courtroom and hates being a part of the criminal justice system. He testified because it was his responsibility to do so, one of the distasteful aspects of the CMHC work.

Warren did a thorough, professional job of examining the defendant and made a persuasive witness on the stand. He testified that the defendant was not insane, but rather self-centered and cruel, with brutal disregard for the rights of others. The defense presented opposing testimony, of course, but Warren was so eloquent, so commonsensical, that his views were the foundation for the defendant's conviction.

Warren took a characteristically perverse pride in being a superb witness. "Anyone can be good at something enjoyable and easy," he said. "But I hate the damn courtrooms, and I hate pompous experts. It was a challenge for me to be a convincing witness and not look like a horses's ass in the process."

After sentencing, the prisoner gave the bailiff a verbal message, which was duly passed along: "You can tell that shrink that he's going to be very, very sorry." The man is now in prison and will be eligible for parole in two years. If he is the person making the threats, who is mailing the notes for him? They have been postmarked from a dozen different postal stations.

The death threats hanging over Warren's family have not only frightened him, they've turned him stubborn, and made him reflective and bitter about psychiatry's evolving position in contemporary society.

As we sit talking over our ritual beer and peanuts, I look at Warren and see Rodin's *The Thinker:* contemplative, hard as granite, and immovable.

"You know me, Marty," he says. "I'm a weird son of a bitch. I don't like running away from anything. I'm afraid for my family, but I'm not going to make any decisions based on fear. I don't want to live my life like that. Call me contrary, obstinate, a nut—anything you want—I'm not going to go into hiding, and I'm not going to give up my job."

Warren talks tough and he is tough, but he's not as tough as he talks. It's true he has stayed with his job, but he does so with less and less conviction as the months go by. One day, after too much beer, he told me that he has taken to scanning medical journals to look for openings elsewhere. Perhaps Alaska, he thinks. Just a little more friction at work and one good offer, and he'll resign in a snap.

He pauses and stares at me intently, eyes smoldering, working the grainy skin over his knuckles, opening and closing his fists: "How many physicians do you know who would stick with this damn job? Would you?"

I shrug. Who's to say? I can't imagine trying to do Warren's job, don't even want to think about it. My cowardice is an old and valued friend, and I sit comfortably with it in my chair as his eyes bore into me.

"Let's try to make some generalizations from this miserable situation," he says. "Let's forget about this particular crazy son of a bitch who wants to kill me. Let's forget about what an abrasive, cantankerous character I am, and let's not even think about what I might have done to have gotten him to hate me. Let's look at the role of a poor goddamn psychiatrist and a poor suffering patient in a CMHC catering to down-and-outers, honky-tonkers, and people just hanging on.

"What keeps a psychiatrist functioning competently in a situation like that?" he asks rhetorically. "The thing that keeps the average reasonably decent psychiatrist doing a decent clinical job is the prospect of helping people. That's baseline for morale. Everything else is layered on top—the money, working conditions—all that stuff takes second place to that feeling of satisfaction which comes from helping patients."

He leans forward, fervent, large index finger peppering the table between us with each burst of words. "But do you know how many patients come to see me because they want anything specifically therapeutic? I'd be surprised if half of them fell into that category. Probably fifty percent are there because they have to see me for some administrative function I can perform.

"Like court-ordered sanity exams. I see lots of those. Like court-ordered competency hearings on borderline senile old people. I see those by the dozens. Like exams to see if people are eligible for aid to the disabled or workmen's compensation. I bet I see a hundred of those in a year. Even some of the people who come in for so-called treatment are there only to go through a ritual: like the drunks who are arrested for driving while intoxicated and are given reduced sentences so long as they are 'in treatment.' Or the junkies, or the petty thieves. It goes on and on and on.

"Those people, they don't regard me as a doctor in any traditional sense. They mostly figure me for an extension of the court, a bureaucratic functionary. They want to see me as briefly as they can, take care of business, and get out. If anything, they are more likely to see me as an obstacle to whatever it is they want rather than as a help. They've got to put on as good a performance as possible so that I'll write something helpful in their record.

"I saw this poor bastard yesterday. He's a working man, a day-laborer at the produce market. He's forty-two years old, and he's been busting his back for twenty-five years already. He's tired and his morale is shot and he's depressed. All he can see ahead of him is twenty more years of fifty-pound sacks and people yelling at him to move faster. He sees no way off the treadmill unless he becomes disabled. His next-door neighbor has back problems and has been adjudged one hundred percent disabled by the V. A. My man says his neighbor makes sixteen hundred dollars per month tax free, not counting side benefits. He tells me none of this crap spontaneously. I have to probe for it, follow my intuition.

"The man comes in to see me, says he has back problems. Says the pain is so bad that he is getting depressed, has even begun to think of suicide. He's already gone to see an orthopedic surgeon, who says some back damage shows up on X-ray. A little bit, but not enough to account for all the trouble he seems to be having. However, there's no objective way of measuring pain. If my man says he's having pain, the orthopedist can't argue with him. What the orthopod will do is say there are findings sufficient to account for partial disability. But partial disability is no good because it's not enough to live on, and it gets reduced in amount if he tries to supplement it by working a little on the side. So if my man wants full disability, he has to see a psychiatrist so he can get partial psychiatric disability to augment his disability from his back.

"So he comes to me, and he is the picture of depression. It's not fake, mind you. It's real enough, but how much of it is related to his back and how much of it is related to his financial problem and the rest of his life situation is anybody's guess. One of his kids is mentally retarded and another kid is an up-and-coming hoodlum, and the man's got problems. He's helping to support his wife's mother, and they live in a lousy building, and he's in debt up to his bellybutton, and he feels trapped. His wife has bad diabetes, and she's barely holding her own.

"Why shouldn't he apply for disability? he figures. He's paid his damn taxes for twenty-five years already. He's entitled to something. He has been a good worker all his life, a reliable family man, and all he's got to show for it are the calluses on his hands, a bad case of hemorrhoids, and the unremitting attentions of several collection agencies.

"Mind you, the man's not a bum. He's not begging. He's got a certain dignity. He simply tells me that he ain't making it, and he ain't gonna make it. The only hope he sees is if he gets disability or if he knocks himself off. He's got a ten-thousand-dollar insurance policy, and that will help support his family for a while at least.

"I don't think he's putting on an act. Maybe he's exaggerating a bit, but who's to know? The point is that he's at the end of his tether. He's depressed, and the best thing I can do to help his depression is help get him declared one hundred percent disabled.

"But where do my loyalties lie? How can you make a so-called medical judgment that is not distorted by personal values? If I write a strong letter in support of disability, I feel like a bleeding heart; and if I write a letter not supporting disability, I feel like an insensitive Calvinist. It all boils down to values, and this poor bastard has to rely on the unknown and inevitably arbitrary biases of a doc he doesn't know and played no part in choosing. I'm assigned to him by the system, and that's where my damn loyalties lie. That's where my paycheck comes from."

"What are you going to do?" I ask.

"Who the hell knows? First, I'm going to go to church and pray for guidance, and then I'll do whatever seems least wrong, and then either way I'll go back to church and confess what I did and pray for forgiveness.

"It used to be that we thought of psychiatric disability as a natural corollary of mental illness, and we viewed 'disability payments as a therapeutic godsend for a disabled soul, an assurance of room and board, which made it possible for people to devote their full energies to working in therapy with us so that they could get better. Now increasingly, I have the sense that the disability payment is becoming an end in itself, and people see me only to give the disability authenticity. Sometimes they see me solely for the purpose of building a legal record, so they can say that they had to start seeing a psychiatrist after some traumatic event at work or a car accident. I see a fair number of patients now who will say, 'Be sure and write in my record that I started having this problem after the forklift accident.' You know exactly what they're doing. They're building a case for some damn personal injury lawyer in the workmen's compensation system.

"This guy with a back pain doesn't really want to be cured. He doesn't want his back pain to go away, and he doesn't want his depression to go away, at least not until he gets his disability settled. Unless he wins the Irish Sweepstakes, his pain and his depression are his only tickets off the loading platform, his only chance for buying a little recreational vehicle and retiring with a fishing pole.

"I can't blame him for giving it a try. Hell, the American dream is early retirement with an assured income and driving off into the sunset. He's taking his only shot at it. The only thing that stands in his way is me. Wonderful basis for a mutually respectful doctor-patient relationship, isn't it? Warren the Healer, they call me. Sprinkling the balm of Gilead on all the pilgrims.

"Shit," he says, and refills his stein from the pitcher. "How many patients like that can you see and still maintain a therapeutic perspective? How much time can you spend with people like that and still have that therapeutic aura about you?

"It's hard enough being therapeutic when the whole system is set up to be therapeutic. When the place in which you work functions like a goddamn eligibility mill in the goddamn governmental bureaucracy, you haven't got a soap bubble's chance in a needle factory.

"Look at it from a truly suffering patient's point of view: he sits in the CMHC waiting room and the guy on his left either will or will not go to jail because of what I say, and the guy on his right either will or will not be declared disabled because of his visit to me. Why should that poor suffering slob in the middle trust me with his innermost conflicts, expose his guilt and fears? How can I develop the kind of trust that I need in a doctor-patient relationship when I spend most of my time processing people to meet the needs of the bureaucracy? Me! For Christ's sake. How the hell did I ever end up in a situation like this?

"You know, Marty, my whole life up to now had led me to a single professional commitment: to helping working-class stiffs who are sick and can't pay for medical or psychiatric care on a fee-for-service basis. It sounds pretentious and self-serving but, damn it, I like being a conscientious doc. But I don't know anyplace I can go without getting all involved in the social control business. Honest to God I don't. I don't see it getting any better in the years ahead, either."

Above our table is one of those cardboard signs, mostly black, with bright red lettering: "NOT RESPONSIBLE FOR PERSONAL ARTICLES." Warren gestures toward it.

"Not responsible. Not responsible. Nobody is clearly responsible to patients any more. It used to be that as doctors we were responsible only to our patients. Now patients are last on the list, after the institution we work for, the state, third-party payers, the board of medical quality assurance, the federal government. God knows who else.

"We've turned into a bunch of cops. Every time the patient turns around, we have to report the fact to some governmental agency. All our discretion is gone. Hell, you of all people ought to know that."

Yes, I know about that. Warren has recalled something that happened to me, and it seems to him to confirm his adversary view of doctor-patient relationships.

I had been working in the emergency room at the time, wearing my general practitioner hat instead of my psychiatrist hat. On this particular day, I was asked to see a three-year-old child who was crying and in obvious pain. She held her right leg very still and clung to her father with both arms. Her grandfather stood watchfully in the background.

I asked what had happened, and the father said that when he had put her to bed, she had suddenly yelled in pain and grabbed her right upper leg. He could think of nothing that might have harmed her. He was upset and solicitous toward his child, yet something about the situation didn't seem right. The nurse on duty and I exchanged glances.

I examined the child and was able to localize the pain fairly well to the right mid-thigh. There was no obvious bruise, and the child seemed to be healthy and otherwise well cared for. I ordered an X-ray.

When the X-ray was completed, it revealed a fracture of the femur—the thigh bone—at mid-shaft, a type of fracture that occurs almost exclusively as the result of a blow from the side. The femur is the most substantial bone in the whole body, like a baseball bat in strength. It does not fracture with trivial force unless it is diseased in some way, and there was no evidence of that in this child. I told the father and grandfather that the girl's leg was broken, and described the necessary treatment. Then I asked the father to come with me. We went to a side room where we could have some privacy, and I said: "Dad, tell me again how this happened."

The man began weeping, with gasping sobs that came from deep within him. He and I spent the next hour together, and as he wept, he told me his story.

He had been upset and impatient. He was a schoolteacher and had been under enormous stress lately. This particular day had been one of the worst. The school overflowed with unruly kids. When he came home, his daughter was cranky and demanding. She started to fuss and then began to scream when he told her to be quiet. He flew into a rage, and told her he was taking her to bed. He hoisted her bodily and, with her kicking and screaming, he slammed her onto her bed. Her upper leg hit the bed rail, and he heard the cracking of her bone.

"I didn't want to hurt her, Doctor," he said. "There's nothing more important to me in the whole world than that little girl." The sobs shook his body. I didn't doubt that he felt guilt and remorse.

The point of my relaying all this here is that I believed the man. However it sounds on paper, in person it had the feel of truth. Yet I understood that corroborative evidence was needed. I reexamined the girl for other signs of abuse, and there were none. I looked through her pediatric chart, and those of the other children in the family, and there were no entries suggestive of mistreatment.

The man said that this was the first time that anything like this had happened, and I believed him. His wife and the wife's father, both solemn and concerned, agreed. He said that if he could have, he would have broken both his own legs to have saved his child such pain. I believed him. He said that such temper tantrums were indulgences that he could not allow himself again, and he volunteered to seek counseling without my suggesting it or urging him. I believed him.

Finally I said that although technically I should report all cases of suspected child abuse to the police, in this case it seemed to me to serve no useful purpose. I was willing to take the responsibility for not reporting it, so long as he and his daughter saw me weekly and I could be confident that both were progressing satisfactorily. In any event, I would need to be seeing the daughter for continued care of her fracture. If ever they should fail to keep an appointment, I would then report him to the police.

He concurred in every regard, as later did his wife and the little girl's grandfather.

Whether my clinical judgment was accurate or not is irrelevant in this situation. If I was clinically in error, it certainly would have been neither the first nor the last time. But, as it turned out, I had no right to use my judgment in deciding whether to report the matter to the police. It was not my place to consider what I thought were the best interests of the child and her father. Their welfare, as assessed by either themselves or by me, was of secondary importance. My primary responsibility was to the institution that employed me, and through it to the state, and to the rules of conduct formulated in the state capital. For if I had been wrong, the liability would not have been mine alone, but the hospital's as well. The hospital therefore could not allow me to base my judgment on the patient's needs as I perceived them. The decision had to be taken out of my hands. So the desk clerk reported to the police that we had treated a patient suspected to be a victim of child abuse, and I was reprimanded.

I've brooded over the matter intermittently for the past several years. "The patient comes first," we were always told in medical school. Who defines what those words mean—and how, operationally, the rule is put into practice? The doctor? The patient?

Warren and I both take long swallows of our beer. He speaks more quietly now. "I don't know who this person is who wants to kill me, but all I can say is I'm not surprised. Maybe he sees me as a double agent, but hell, I *am* a double agent. I like to see myself working for the patient's benefit, but half of what I do is specifically geared to bureaucratic needs, whether the patient benefits or not.

"The thing that bothers me is that there are a lot of needy people out there—call them sick, call them sufferers, call them whatever you like—and they need reasonably compassionate and competent people to help them. This adversary flavor turns people away from seeking treatment and dissuades doctors from going to the folks who may need them the most.

"This death threat to me simply dramatizes the whole adversary thing and makes me fear my patients as much as some of them fear me. The whole thing stinks. I wish I could find the son of a bitch who hates me so much and try to explain the whole goddamn thing to him. We're both victims, I'd tell him. I don't hate him and I don't want to kill him, but I will if I have to. We're at war. Doctors and patients have gotten sucked into a war where too often we are on opposite sides. Our interests diverge. I hate it, but I don't know what else to do. Do you?"

It's been almost a year now since I last saw Warren. Sooner or later, one of us will call the other. Somehow I hold back. There are dozens of explanations, but one is inescapable for me: I find his views on the war between doctors and patients to be extremely disquieting. Flawed and simplistic though they are, they have enough truth so that I can't dismiss them entirely.

Warren's clinical ability is a casualty of the war as he envisions it. Though not an entirely innocent victim, he is now functioning clinically at a far lower level than his natural talent would ordinarily allow. Because he has come to see himself as a frequent adversary of his patients, he is not always the healer that he could be, and that so many of his patients need. He has lost something sacred in the process, and so have his patients. Warren's dream of being the quintessence of compassion to his workingman patients hasn't come true. His compassion is a combustible commodity, and it incinerates to ashes in the cold blue flame of anger.

And for what? Warren serves a function in the criminal justice system, civil court proceedings, and our nation's workmen's compensation process. Do the contributions he makes in these areas make up for the loss of his therapeutic morale? For the loss of his helpfulness to patients? Are they worth it? And if so, worth it to whom?

13 THE DOCTOR-PATIENT RELATIONSHIP: Conflicting Allegiances

Sometimes people talk about doctors—and we talk about ourselves—as though we were creatures apart. That separateness, once based on importance and esteem, is now often adversarial, rooted in the implication that physicians are unable to understand the process of health care as seen through patients' eyes, that our interests and values are different, and often not in our patients' welfare.

Over the years, I have seen my role—and patients' perception of that role—change qualitatively. More and more often, patients whom I meet for the first time approach their contact with me with a set of attitudes and expectations that makes my task of helping them more complicated and less pleasant. Unknown physicians face suspicion, wariness, sometimes outright hostility, and a relentlessly questioning manner from new patients who appear for treatment.

Who can blame these patients? I have been a patient myself on many occasions, and I've had several major surgical procedures. I've waited anxiously for the biopsy report to come back, reporting on tissues taken from my own body, with the gnawing emptiness which comes from the possibility that one's life hangs in the balance. I've watched people I love struggle with the implications and effects of serious illness, and I understand at a deeply personal level that the doctor's traditional position of power creates a potential for good and for ill.

Patients worry about being abused at the hands of the health-care system—and people like me—and their concerns are far too frequently justified. Yet where does that leave me, a reasonably conscientious doctor trying to do a reasonably conscientious job? Each time I see a new patient, I expect to have to start from a defensive position, working hard in the brief period of time allotted to me to develop a relationship based on mutual trust—yet simultaneously aware that the patient's reluctance to trust is based on realistic concerns.

Patients sense the potential for undesirable consequences and act accordingly: they approach the doctor expecting that in some minor or major way the contact will lead to grief—the services will cost too much, drug side effects and diagnostic and therapeutic adventures will lead to physical dangers, or the cool impersonality of the doctor in the "therapeutic setting" will lead to dehumanization.

What patients tend not to perceive, yet what I feel keenly to be an equal or greater factor in the breach between doctor and patient, is the ominous role of rules and guidelines which derive from often distant third parties. In each setting where I have seen patients, now and in the past, I have been struck by how much of my time is spent performing essentially administrative, quasi-legal functions, with therapeutic components minimal or absent.

A representative though seemingly trivial example concerns a patient needing a return-to-work slip. A woman working at a nearby automotive assembly plant caught a cold and decided to stay home for several days, treating herself with an appropriate self-care regimen. However, in order to qualify for sick leave for the time spent away from work, she needed to present evidence that she had seen a physician. Therefore, when she was ready to return to work she came to the drop-in medical clinic. Perhaps she tried to get an appointment with her own physician, assuming she had one; but frequently in bureaucratic medical settings a patient must make nonemergency appointments with her regular doctor weeks in advance. The drop-in clinic is by definition run on a nonappointment basis, and she had to wait a couple of hours before getting to see me—because there were a lot of other people in the same boat as she, and patients with more urgent problems kept getting moved up to the front of the line.

Finally she saw me. Of course she was angry. She had waited a couple of hours, and all she needed was a signature. I didn't have to examine her, or treat her in any way. I simply had to sign a slip saying that she had seen a physician. I had become an obstacle to what she felt was rightfully hers: her sick leave. She felt ripped off by the system and angry at me personally as its representative. As I turned to go, she muttered just loud enough for me to hear: "Damn doctors."

For my part, the contact was equally unsavory. Who wants to spend a working day encountering angry people who blame you in part for their misery? The encounter becomes even less satisfying because it represents an enormous waste of talent and training. Did I become a doctor for this?

In this homely example—which is repeated in principle many times each week in my meetings with patients—lies the essence of a growing and as yet poorly recognized aspect of contemporary health care. The doctor-patient relationship has become so encumbered with other demands that the therapeutic aspect has often come to be peripheral.

It's important to understand that even as the patient feels dehumanized, so does the doctor. As I feel my own uniqueness blurred, as my judgment is less important, and as I am less confident of my own integrity, it's harder for me to impart individualized care to the patients I see. As I meet each new patient, I always take care to introduce myself by name. Even though we all wear name tags, I'm frequently struck by how few patients remember the name of the last physician they saw in the clinic, and I find myself wondering, will this person remember my name in a week or even in a few hours? Or be able to distinguish me from the waiter or supermarket cashier who provided services yesterday?

A growing percentage of patients now come to the clinic not expecting or even wanting to develop rapport. What they want is a technical service, given with reasonable competence and efficiency, and without any fuss. Some are nice about it and some are demanding: examine my eyes, prescribe penicillin for my cold, sign my work slip, sign my insurance physical, give me a tetanus shot, sew up my wound. More and more of them know exactly what they want, and the identity of the physician who provides the services is incidental. From their point of view, their attitude makes perfect sense.

Under the circumstances, I try to remain pleasant, but too frequently it is the wary, antiseptic courtesy of a clerk in a busy department store.

What worries me even more—and what is deeply unsettling to many thoughtful physicians—is that much of what we do, or are asked to do, is manifestly not in our patients' best interests. We order tests which instinct and medical judgment suggest are inappropriate, yet which adherence to legal and administrative standards seems to require. Patients are, after all, increasingly strangers, and it is better to be safe than sorry—safety is too often evaluated on the basis of minimizing disruption or complaints or lawsuits. I call it acquiescent medicine. Whatever the patient wants, he or she can have. I don't think you need an X-ray for this condition, but if you say you want it and I can't talk you out of it easily, I'll order it for you. It's easier and less hazardous to me to do so. I think penicillin for your common cold will do you more harm than good, but if you disagree with me, I'll prescribe it for you nevertheless. It's your body, and the choice is up to you. I've got a waiting room full of patients to see, and I haven't got time to argue.

Nor is it only the patient who asks us to do things that, in our judgment, may be harmful. The "guardians" of the patients' welfare do so as well. My personal struggle with the situation in which child abuse occurred is simply one example, but there are many others in which the doctor is compelled by law to report certain conditions, diagnoses, and events to authorities. The patient who has a lapse in consciousness must be reported to the Department of Motor Vehicles. The patient whom I perceive as being unable to provide for his or her own food, clothing, or shelter must be detained—involuntarily if necessary—for evaluation at a designated institution. The patient who has any one of a variety of infectious diseases, including mumps and measles, must be reported to the appropriate department of our state government.

In the interests of informed consent, perhaps we should place signs in all medical offices, clinics, and hospitals declaring: "Before you enter these doors, you should know that if you have any of the following conditions, your doctor will be required by law to report you to the appropriate authorities . . ."

All of these laws have evolved for sensible enough reasons—and stem from the generally beneficent intent of their sponsors—but unfortunately they require me to behave in a way that often makes me feel I'm in an adversary relationship to my patients. The laws compel me to sacrifice my primary obligation to the patient and to the confidentiality of communications between us, in favor of bureaucratic implementation of the public welfare. Consequently, when I can do so without putting myself in undue jeopardy, I often ignore such legal obligations.

When I see a person who has what appears to be gonorrhea, I am supposed to report the matter to the Department of Health. I understand the reasoning behind the requirement: the report enables people working in the health department to track down all possible sexual contacts of my patients, to advise them that they have been exposed to gonorrhea, and to encourage them to seek treatment. As a matter of actual practice, however, I only report the gonorrhea if the presence of the disease has been documented by laboratory test, in which case my failure to report—an indictable crime—would be supported by concrete evidence. If I merely presume the gonorrhea is present, because the urethral discharge and the pattern of onset of the problem are typical, I treat the patient with the appropriate antibiotic without filing an official report. Instead, I tell the patient: "It's *your* responsibility to tell your sexual contacts of their exposure to this disease. If you fail to do so, they will suffer from your lack of responsibility; and it will be the price they pay for their selection of you as a lover."

In taking this approach, I recognize that I am in violation of the law and vulnerable to prosecution if I am apprehended. I could even be deprived of my license to practice medicine. Only recently a California physician's license was suspended for failure to report a case of hepatitis in a food service worker. I further understand that infectious disease specialists and epidemiologists will think my behavior reprehensible. They believe that the public good must supersede platitudes about individual responsibility and the sanctity of the doctor-patient relationship. Yet I behave as I do because my actions help to reaffirm a fundamental though tarnished value: my first responsibility as a physician is to my patient. When I make mistakes, I tell myself, let them be in the interest of the patient and the patient's right to self-determination. I will behave responsibly to the patient, and give the patient the opportunity to behave responsibly to himself and to society.

The doctor-patient relationship is under enormous strain these days. Each physician must daily confront the issue of allegiances. To what degree am I responsible to each of the following: the government, third-party insurers, the institution in which I work, my co-workers, my patient, the patient's family? Each of us makes decisions and compromises, yet at some point each must draw the line and say: "To continue to compromise in these specific ways will so brutalize my conception of my proper role that I could not continue and respect my own behavior." The choice is an individual one, but of course there are patterns. I know I am not alone in my response to the infectious disease reporting requirements.

In the mid-1970s the California Supreme Court handed down the Tarasoff decision, holding that if a physician, during the course of professional activities, comes to the conclusion that a given patient is dangerous to a third party, the physician has a duty to warn that third party of the danger. On the face of it, the decision seems fair and in accord with the general public good. However, there are aspects to the decision that make me very uncomfortable. The doctor has been placed under special jeopardy, and the doctor-patient relationship has been used for special purposes. If I as a neighbor or acquaintance learn that someone may be dangerous, I am under no special obligation to warn a third party—but if I obtain the same information in my capacity as a physician, then I am obligated to do so, or face criminal charges. The doctor-patient relationship has accumulated yet another entry in a growing list of police functions.

I have no objection to protecting the public. In fact, the converse is true: as a citizen I feel my responsibilities keenly. I am disturbed, however, when the state takes advantage of the privacy accorded me by my patients to *require* me to act in what it sees as the public interest. As an individual physician, my only choice is to comply or not to comply with the laws as they affect me. The laws themselves derive from a level of decision-making to which I have no access. If discussion at that level faced the underlying concepts which lead to such legislation, the speakers would deal explicitly with the appropriateness of using the medical profession as an instrument of social control.

Thomas Szasz broached the issue in the mid-1950s and carried the torch almost single-handedly for many years, but he now has many spirited followers. His point then, and as it has evolved over the years, was this: illness, and especially mental illness, is a metaphor for socially undesirable behavior; and health, especially mental health, is a metaphor for socially acceptable behavior. The physician's role, therefore, is to conceal conflict and deviance as illness, and to redefine pacification, brainwashing, and warehousing as treatment.

Most of us didn't believe Szasz's strident rhetoric when he began, but times are changing and we are beginning to feel the implications of his observations on our own practices. Despite their oversimplifications, the cogency of his arguments has accumulated more and more adherents as various media presentations have brought to light instances of physical and mental abuse of psychiatric patients in institutions, and the blatantly political use of psychiatry in the Soviet Union. There are numerous popular plays, books, and movies that have portrayed "treatment" in the same way—i.e., as simply a metaphor for the oppression of individuality.

The heightened consciousness of various ethnic groups has led them to trumpet a similar message from their various perspectives. Ardent feminists say that psychiatry is simply a sexist means of subduing female aspirations for equality by labeling female assertiveness as castrating or neurotic behavior. Outspoken blacks say psychiatry functions as an elitist, predominantly white middle-class ideology for suppression of unique black cultural values. Homosexuals vigorously protested being labeled as mentally disordered—"Stop it, you're making me sick," said one group—and succeeded in a campaign within the American Psychiatric Association to have the "diagnosis" of homosexuality removed from the list of mental disorders.

Where does that leave the physician? I thought I had entered this profession to be helpful to people called patients. I had no conscious awareness—and have none now—of any desire to impose my values on others, to use my part in the doctor-patient relationship as a means of oppressing others, or to serve the state or bureaucratic institutions in opposition to the interests of my patients.

But Szasz's criticisms strike close to the bone, and I see the situation growing worse rather than better. In order to serve the many rather than the few, more and more physicians are practicing, like myself, in bureaucratized settings. The impersonal clinic is going to play a greater role in future medical care, not a lesser one; and private practitioners are also subject to regulations that restrict and constrict their daily interactions with patients. No physician is immune to the multiplying entanglements of the regulatory apparatus. Increasingly it will be the state that determines what a doctor does and does not do with patients.

Szasz says: "I particularly hope that Americans in increasing numbers will begin to discriminate between two types of physicians: those who heal, not so much because they are saints, but because that is their *job;* and those who harm, not because they are sinners, but because that is their *job* [his italics]. And if some doctors harm—torture rather than treat, murder the soul rather than minister to the body—that is, in part, because society, the state, asks them, and pays them, to do so."

Where will my patients see me in that dichotomy? Where will I see myself?

I am also concerned about something which Szasz didn't stress—that the system distorts the patients even as it distorts the doctors: the system produces a certain kind of sufferer even as it produces a certain kind of healer. Some people come to doctors for healing, not so much because they are saints but because they have few acceptable alternatives; and some come to doctors for processing, not so much because they are sinners but because the system leaves them few acceptable alternatives. We are all in this together.

I am pessimistic about what the future holds for conscientious physicians who attempt to confront complicated human problems in a clinical setting. Everyone seems to know what's wrong with health care except the people who actually take care of patients, who are thought to be too self-interested to be trusted.

In the hospital rooms and corridors, in the clinics and consulting rooms, in the offices and at the bedsides—the clinicians of this country are struggling, most of them conscientiously, to be of some help to an endless stream of sufferers. The work can be not only physically exhausting, but emotionally exhausting too. Our health-care system should be making their job easier, but it's not. The system too often grinds down clinicians, leaching out their humanity and making dust of their therapeutic zeal.

Is it any wonder that contemporary physicians often feel the temptation to flee from their patients?

14 ROSE: The Doctor with No Patients

When Rose finished her psychiatric training in the late 1960s, there was no question about what she would do with her skills: she would take them to the inner-city areas where so many residents had been neglected by traditional private practice approaches.

She could have gone anywhere. As a highly credentialed black woman, at a time of ethnic consciousness and rising feminism, the labels made her attractive to many universities, even gave her premature access to high-level policy-making positions in state and federal government. However, the same cultural forces that created these opportunities also helped influence Rose to spend her time as a clinician for the people who needed her. Underserved is what they were called, and underserved is how Rose thought of them.

"Baby," she says a dozen years later, "I was so wet behind the ears that you couldn't have dried me out with a twelve-to-one martini. I was so sure of my own ability to help people I would have volunteered to be a psychiatrist in Dante's Inferno." She wasn't the only one, of course. A lot of people were naïve.

Rose went to work in an urban ghetto, in a community mental health center (CMHC) designed to serve over two hundred thousand residents of the city's one million population. Lots of them were blacks, but there were other people too—Latinos, Asians, American Indians, whites. The one thing her patients had in common was their persisting poverty. No money, no resources, no prospects. It seemed to all her friends, including me, that she had picked a pretty gruesome place to work.

Rose loved it for a while.

She started with the zest that is her trademark: always enthusiastic, always helpful, always cordial and thoughtful. Patients flocked to her. "I saw so many patients," she says, spreading her arms to encompass the world, "it was like somebody was sending organized tours through my office. Like none of God's children could get to heaven without first stopping to see Mama Rose."

Early on, she discovered that patients in her community did not like to make or keep appointments, so she decided to run her practice open-house style. From early morning until she left in the evening, there were always people waiting on the rows of clinic chairs outside her door. Simple people and complicated people, sad or angry, worn out or doped up or crazy—they all came to see Rose.

Some were talkative and some not, but most seemed to derive comfort from her mere presence. For them, Rose provided a reliable haven and an authoritative perspective from which they could gather the strength to struggle with their unending travails. Sometimes it was difficult to know even where to begin. "The people I see don't have problems; they've got messes," she said.

What many of the patients who came to see Rose wanted was compassion and understanding. Everybody was compassion-deprived.

"There's so little tenderness in the big city," Rose would say. "People come to the psychiatrist in the hope of getting their tenderness tanks topped off. Person after person comes in asking for love and understanding, figuring that's what I'm there for. And that's how I conceive of my role too, at least in part. After the eighth or fifteenth needy person each and every day, though, I find myself getting resentful. I'm supposed to give tenderness, but I get relatively little back in return. People are self-absorbed but expect me not to be. They come in irritated by the bureaucratic procedures and dump a little of their aggravation on my head, expecting me to somehow be immune to similar feelings and behavior.

"In some ways, it's a setup for resentment on the psychiatrist's part. You're supposed to—and do by and large—care more about individual patients than they do about you. They've got troubles of their own and don't come to the doctor to have to worry about the doctor. The salaries we get are supposed to be compensation enough. Sometimes, I need compassion and understanding from the patients in return, but I feel guilty asking for it, since I'm getting paid and they are not."

So Rose struggled to find alternative ways of plying her psychiatric skills, ones which were less costly to her own emotional reserves yet provided a useful service. That's how her flight from patients started.

At first she began doing a few hours of administrative work each week, "just as a change of pace." She was appointed to the mayor's committee on drug abuse. What if she didn't see any patients during those hours? It was stimulating and it got her out of the clinic, and she thought she was doing something of value.

She started developing new approaches to treatment too. Because of the constant press of patients and because it made practical sense, Rose began seeing patients with similar problems in groups: alcoholic men, adolescents with sexual troubles, obese women, people with stress-related physical ailments like ulcers, and lots of depressed people.

Depression was rampant. Her patients viewed the world as an inhospitable place, often cruel and unyielding. Families felt trapped by miserable slum housing. Adolescent girls were trapped by ignorance and their fertile wombs. Boys were trapped by drugs and gangs and violence. Men were trapped by dead-end jobs, macho expectations, and a sense of failure. And the women. Rose ached for the women; she could identify with them so easily.

Some people liked the groups because they gave members an opportunity to share experiences to see their problems weren't unique, to help one another through mutual support. But the intimacy of the doctor-patient relationship was diluted, and many of the patients were unhappy about that. Rose felt restless. She missed that rare and exclusive bond which can form between a patient who is really needy and a doctor who really cares, when the two struggle together in private.

Rose was keenly aware of her own ambivalence. She wanted the reciprocal intimacy of the ideal doctor-patient relationship, but she was reluctant to expend energy in many nonreciprocal relationships in order to find one or two that were truly satisfying. And there just seemed to be too many people in need to see all of them individually, and their depression was too contagious.

The groups proved to be expedient. If Rose could see a dozen people per hour instead of one or a few, the waiting list would be cut to nothing and the clinic's "patients-seen statistics" would improve considerably. The more patients seen in the clinic, the greater the financial support likely to come from the federal government. Rose's boss, the clinic's administrator, a nonphysician with a master's degree in health-care administration, encouraged her to see people in groups whenever possible.

The most successful groups in terms of numbers were the medication groups. "Medication patients" in Rose's clinic were people who had been coming for treatment for some time and had reached a plateau where further time-consuming counseling or psychotherapy either seemed fruitless or not cost effective from the clinic's point of view. The patients therefore came to the clinic primarily for prescription refills, and sometimes for a doctor's signature to certify that they were under a physician's care. Such statements were often required by a probation officer or school principal or employer or other interested party.

Each visit followed a consistent pattern:

"How are you doing?"

"Okay."

"Is the medication helping you?"

"Yes."

"Shall I give you another month's supply?"

"Please."

"Okay. Here's the prescription. See you in a month."

If there were any complications, such as side effects from the medication, the visit might take as long as ten minutes, but the vast majority could be completed in as little as two minutes. Rose even managed to speed up the process further by having the receptionist type up the prescriptions and simply seeing the patient long enough to affix her signature.

Once, when she and I talked about the medication groups, I kidded her about merchandising pill-pushing and suggested that she could be replaced by one of those candy machines they have in the clinic coffee shop without any loss of intimacy. The machine could be com-

puter operated so that the patient could insert a Medicaid card and
get back a prescription refill without ever having to see a physician.

She didn't think this was funny: "Listen, Smarty Marty, if you
think you can do it better, I know I can find a job for you right here."

I shut up, but I had struck a nerve.

While the medication production lines filled a clear administrative
need, they gave Rose no personal gratification. She rationalized that
she was performing a useful service but realized that her considerable
clinical skill was going to waste. She was feeling less and less like a
physician, and this eroded her self-respect. She decided she would try
to see some psychotherapy patients each week in addition to the
medication patients, even if time pressures limited their number. She
was getting increasingly involved in medical politics, and time was at
a premium. She was on the governor's health advisory committee
now, and on several national committees on minority health issues.

She looked around for suitable psychotherapy candidates, meaning
persons who were bright, verbal, insightful, willing to make a commitment to probing the inner workings of the mind, and able to make
time available for doing so. People who would not only respond to
Rose's therapeutic skills, but who would also understand and appreciate Rose's craftsmanship. People who would contribute proportionately to building a really solid doctor-patient relationship.

In searching for such uniquely introspective and giving persons
among a population generally much more preoccupied with their
problems in the external world, Rose had no illusions. She was looking for psychotherapy patients because she needed to reassure herself
that she was still able to perform a skill that was central to her own
identity as a clinician.

Unfortunately for her, she encountered enormous competition for
"good psychotherapy candidates" at the center. The many people
who regarded themselves as psychotherapists—the nurse, social
worker, psychologist, and others—hungered for such patients too,
and none of those who screened new patients would refer to her the
kinds of patients she wanted. They kept the "good ones" for themselves. She laughs about in in retrospect: "It was like everyone was
maneuvering to pick the cashews out of a bowl of mixed nuts, and
Rose was the last to get her hand in."

And once she did find satisfactory patients, her own attendance at
their sessions was not sufficiently reliable for her to be very helpful.

There were always things coming up: an emergency budget committee meeting, a policy session with the mayor, an urgent conclave with
the governor's advisory group. One day she sat down and reflected
that the only psychotherapy patients who continued seeing her were
the ones who were well enough not really to need her.

She became increasingly listless. Most of her workday hours were
spent with medication patients or doing administrative chores or supervising the clinical work of nonpsychiatrists at the center. She
found this last chore especially ironic: she who was seeing so few therapy patients, sometimes none at all, supervising the activities of others who were doing that for which she had been arduously trained.

She was a good supervisor, her co-workers told her: wise and insightful and helpful in her suggestions. But she felt her role lacked
authenticity. Not only was she not doing what she was telling others
to do, but she was beginning to have serious misgivings about her so-
called position of authority in relation to other professionals.

Practically speaking, hers was a position of influence rather than
authority. Though officially she was clinical supervisor of other nonpsychiatric professionals, and was developing a national reputation as
an expert in several areas, in actual practice she could not order anyone to do anything.

On one occasion, I visited her in her office and she gave me an example. "Take that patient over there." She nodded toward a woman
as we walked through an occupational therapy area toward Rose's office. The woman, who was leaning against a mauve concrete wall,
wore a dirty white sweater and a pair of bright green polyester slacks
stretched across her large belly. Her skin was dark and her hair unkempt.

"That poor woman came to the clinic three days ago," Rose continued. "She arrived totally decompensated. Her husband is an alcoholic
and beats her. Her oldest son is in prison. Her younger son is a fla-
grant transvestite and heroin addict. Her teenage daughter ran away
from home five months ago and hasn't been heard from since. As if
that weren't enough reason to be depressed, the final straw came
when her little poodle was poisoned by some neighborhood sadist.
The poor thing came in here nearly hysterical, hopeless, hearing the
voice of her own deceased mother telling her what a rotten person she
is.

"We tried to get her into the state hospital, but it's filled to capacity and is not accepting any new patients. So we tried to treat her here. There are a thousand ways of treating her. We can give her medications, we can give her individual psychotherapy or group psychotherapy or marital counseling. We can do anything or we can do nothing. No matter what, she's probably going to start feeling a little better in time just because she is spending days away from her crazy home. The problem here is that no one person can decide what approach to take. We have to negotiate a treatment plan.

"With that woman, I thought some medication would be helpful. I don't think it's the only treatment, but it's a useful part of the treatment. Her life is so screwed up that there is no magic potion which will turn her zoo of a home into a Garden of Eden, but I think it would help give her an edge to make coping just a little easier. So I suggested medication to her primary therapist, who in this case happens to be a nurse.

"But the nurse didn't think she should have medication. She believes doctors prescribe too much medicine. I agree, but I think that I can make a reasonable case for giving *this* woman some pills. The nurse thinks I'm wrong.

"What do I do? If I bawl out the nurse, she'll call me authoritarian and rude, and I'll never get anything done around here. I can't fire her, because in spite of the fact that I'm supervising psychiatrist and ultimately responsible for what goes on here, the nurse doesn't work for me, she works for the nursing service."

Rose closed her office door to give us some privacy before continuing: "Throughout the entire city health system, in the clinics and hospitals, on the surgical service, on the cardiac care unit, everywhere, the nurses are administratively under the control of the director of nurses. If I have a complaint about a nurse, I talk to my supervisor who will talk to a nursing supervisor, and the two of them will call in the nurse and myself, and we will discuss interpersonal problem-solving strategies to iron out our mutual differences.

"Now suppose I think that the social worker should meet with the patient's family. The woman's got a disastrous family situation, and it would be helpful to get a better sense of what they are like as people, and what things look like from their point of view. So I ask the social worker to do that, but she says she has this meeting to go to, some administrative tasks to look after, and those other patients to see, and she won't be able to get to my patient's family till next week.

So I say that in my judgment seeing this family should take priority. But it doesn't work that way. She says she is a co-equal professional, capable of establishing priorities on her own, and she will decide in what order things must be done. She works administratively under the division of social service, and if I have any complaints, I have to have my boss talk to her boss.

"The same thing happens again and again, with the occupational therapist, the psychologist, everyone right down the line. There's no such thing as a single chain of command. There are dozens of chains of command. If you want to get anything done, you can't *tell* people what to do, you've got to *convince* them.

"Physicians no longer have unquestioned authority in health matters. Nobody has unquestioned authority. In theory, this clinic and the whole city health system is being run on an interdisciplinary team approach. The idea is that no one person, no one discipline, can do it alone. But it's not really interdisciplinary, it's multidisciplinary. Everybody too often is pulling in different directions. Sometimes I think, Multidisciplinary, hell. They're planning to take over. They'll just hire us physicians to work as technicians, to write prescriptions, and to keep around as scapegoats when things go wrong. Everybody wants to practice medicine without a license."

About six months after our conversation, Rose quit her job at the CMHC and took an administrative post with the state health department. She no longer sees any patients.

She and I have since talked about the quandary of the clinician in institutional settings in considerable detail. "What is going to keep good clinicians involved in patient care?" she says. "Especially with the neediest and most underserved patients? The work is so hard and intrinsically unrewarding. If you want any of the conventional rewards of prestige, money, and personal comfort, you have to look elsewhere.

"When I was putting in sixteen hours a day at the CMHC taking care of patients," she says, "I had a few splashy successes, but mostly I busted my back with no tangible results. The patients were like lightbulbs: as long as I was generating the energy, they would glow a little bit—but if I slacked off, their spark of light would flicker and they would return to their natural depleted state. Everybody thought that I was so vital and enthusiastic at work, but I'd come home and weep for hours. I got so discouraged, it was as if I was at the bottom of a well, and the walls kept getting higher and more slippery, and I just panicked and decided I had to get out before I forgot what the sunshine was like. Every now and then you meet a patient who brightens your day, who tries to give a little something in return. But most of the patients just suck you dry.

"The CMHC where I worked was just a bummer. Everybody was depressed, even the patients. All the employees who worked there for more than a couple of years were burned out. The staff treated the psychotic patients, and I treated the neurotic staff. At least I had the long-suffering staff to insulate me from the patients. The folks who had most contact with patients day in and day out were the people with the least training, the least prestigious titles, and the smallest salaries. I don't see how they could stand it.

"I ran to politics and administration not only because I thought it was the practical thing to do, but because I was getting overwhelmed by the burdens of patient care and staff care. And of course I enjoy meeting all those fancy people, participating in decisions that involve hundreds of thousands, even millions, of dollars. I enjoy reading about myself in the papers. Lecturer. Policy maker. Expert. Making pronouncements about this or that. I do feel guilty about leaving patient care—but I don't have the guts to go back. It took too much out of me, and the rewards available in other directions are too great."

As she shakes her head back and forth somberly, a strand of curly black hair detaches itself from her right temple and swings over her right eye. She reaches up, winding the filaments about her fingers, winding and unwinding as she muses: "You know, in medical school they thought I was going to be a great doctor. In internship I received a special award for being a compassionate and dedicated clinician. Now I find that as a clinician, I've burned out. I've got more tenacity and energy than most people I know, and I've burned out. How the hell do all the docs manage to stay on the firing line, day in and day out? How do they do it?"

We're silent for a long time, two old friends brooding together in silence.

"And you," she says. "How about you?"

"What about me?"

"How many patients are you seeing in therapy these days?"

"Not any," I say, a familiar constriction starting up in my chest.

She smiles at me: "How come?" The question is so soft that it's barely a whisper.

"I haven't got it in me now. Taking care of patients on an intimate long-term basis demands more than I have to give." The words taste like plaster in my mouth.

I keep feeling I *should* be doing psychotherapy. I *should* be seeing individual patients in a developing relationship over time. I *should* have the emotional energy to sustain patients over the long haul. Isn't that what being a doctor is all about?

"You're teaching now?" she asks.

I nod.

"Teaching medical students about the doctor-patient relationship?"

I nod again.

"Doesn't that strike you as a bit ironic?"

What can I say? Of course it's ironic.

We sit quietly once more. I have no notion of what she is thinking. I'm thirsty. I want to go off someplace and be by myself. Maybe Rose senses my thoughts. She stands up to go, then leans over to kiss me on the cheek.

"Cheer up, sweetie," she says. "We aren't alone. I'll bet there are hundreds, maybe thousands, of docs who are struggling with the same issues at this very moment."

Terrific. That's all this world needs. More burned-out doctors.

Who's going to take care of the patients?

15 THE END OF "THE DOCTOR KNOWS BEST"

For half a century, medicine provided a wellspring for some of our nation's finest and most dramatic achievements. The field, viewed with only a little charity, embodied our most cherished ideals: the can-do spirit, combined with ingenuity, organization, and self-sacrifice, leading to eventual triumph over adversity. The democratic humanitarianism which, while selfless in motivation, nonetheless enriched the performers of blessed miracles. The doctor and nurse drama, the quintessential American romance, man and woman joined together in an idealistic quest, who, in doing good deeds, win the love and respect of the community, and the house on the hill as well. Nor was it simply a fantasy. The myth had some substance, and the substance exuded an intoxicating scent that seduced the nation—and physicians as well.

In the first fifty years of this century, the excitement of being a physician permeated the medical profession. The public's imagination was exhilarated by developments in infectious disease prevention, control, and treatment. Illnesses that had been scourges of mankind for centuries were apparently wiped out as public health problems: yellow fever, plague, tuberculosis, and poliomyelitis. "To have lived through a revolution," said Osler, "to have seen a new birth of science, a new dispensation of health, to reorganize medical schools, remodel hospitals, a new outlook for humanity, is not given to every generation." Those days were "so full of happiness, so full of hope"; and the average practitioner sensed the spirit and basked in the reflected glow of public admiration generated by the dramatic events of the time.

As one impossible achievement was piled upon another, we began to take it for granted that every medical problem was potentially solvable—whether it was transplanting organs from one body to another, creating life from genetic soup, or providing standardized, compassionate health care for all our citizens.

When it seemed that medicine's destiny was to solve all the problems to which it devoted its full attention, citizens became increasingly amenable to defining new problems in medical terms. Many came to believe that health care, broadly conceived and efficiently distributed, could resolve all society's ills: poverty, prejudice, ignorance, crime, and more. Research in mental retardation revealed that some people who had heretofore been regarded as hopeless idiots could become essentially normal citizens if appropriate preventative or therapeutic measures were taken. Poverty and disease were shown to be intimately intertwined; if we could cure the latter, might we not remedy the former? Even crime seemed to be the product of unenlightened child upbringing, the malevolent effects of which might respond to proper pediatric and psychiatric attention, if only we allocated our resources sensibly.

Political reformers were quick to take advantage of medicine's popularity and learned to redefine their own special interests and projects in medical terms. One savvy leader, in organizing a revolutionary approach to rural poverty in the South, cautioned his followers who hadn't yet learned the appropriate rhetoric: "If you want to achieve the successes of the Red Guard, learn to behave like the Red Cross." The program overcame local conservative opposition to food stamps by having a physician *prescribe* groceries as a treatment for what was said to be a bona fide medical condition: malnutrition among all the blacks in the county.

Medicine often fostered such values and profited from them; but, as in so many things, the seduction was mutual. With both wanting desperately to believe, the doctor has said to the patient: "Believe in me. Believe in my concepts or my methods, and I will enhance the general quality of your life, your productivity, and your happiness." And the patient, in a willing and grateful suspension of disbelief, said: "You're the doctor. The doctor knows best."

Any human problem became an appropriate target of the physician's expertise. Are you fighting with your spouse? Talk to your doctor. Is your teenager incorrigible? Talk to your doctor. Are you burdened by strain on your job? Get a note from your doctor. Do you want to be exempt from the military draft? Find an M. D. who will be your ally.

As mundane problems like these gradually became a part of the doctor's purview, a subtle shift in American values accompanied the process. The growing belief was that suffering need no longer be a fact of life. Discomfort could be relieved rather than endured. Stoicism seemed outdated, antithetical to current realities, certainly foolish, and perhaps even—dare we say it?—"sick." Anything that was sick was bad, even reprehensible, and vice versa. *Sick* replaced *evil* and *sinful* in the American vocabulary; and *healthy* became the most desirable of adjectives to be applied to practically anything: motivation, relationships, behavior, thought, even entire societies. Anything that could be treated should be treated; and if the individual couldn't afford the financial cost, then the community would pick up the tab.

The general welfare of society came to be equated with optimum health, so that "unnecessary" deviations from optimum health anywhere were seen as blots on the nation's conception of itself. Increasingly health, as a societal metaphor, superseded other traditional American values, even freedom of choice. Health *care* in itself came to be a fundamental American value, even a right, to be guaranteed by governmental action. People who protested public health programs such as immunization requirements, pasteurized milk, iodized salt, or fluoridated water were regarded as kooks. Nothing was more important than the health of our people, they were told. Individual choice had to yield to the public good.

Expectations were layered upon expectations. If health was to be the rubric for all that was good, and health care was the vehicle for delivering it, then the American people expected, in the democratic tradition, universally available health care and, in the competitive scientific tradition, high technologic performance with minimum possible error. There were to be no second-class recipients, and no second-class purveyors of care.

Yet many groups, for their own diverse reasons, pointed out that the expectations were hardly consistent with reality. Many people "in need of services" did not get them. Poor people and ethnic minorities did not have the same access to services as did those more favored. Surveys by the score showed that the nation overflowed with "hidden diabetics" and "hidden hypertensives" and large numbers of people "needing" psychiatric services to which they had no access. Worse, some of the people who had access to such services didn't utilize them, or, if they did, received no improvement from them. And so the rhetoric became even more ambitious and hopeful: if only we could develop some outreach services, bring health care to those who lacked either the wit or ability to seek it on their own. If only we could make all practitioners as knowledgeable and skilled as they have the potential to be. If only we could organize the whole mass of needs and services and recipients and purveyors into one coherent organized system—an integrated health-care system—*then* our nation would be healthy and our healthy nation would inevitably be a happy one.

And that's what we have supposedly been building: an integrated health-care system, nationwide, which represents the fulfillment of all our inflated expectations as a people and our growing sense of entitlement as individuals. The result has been so dramatic as to revolutionize the nature and emotional climate of medical practice in a mere score of years.

It's impossible to talk about what has happened and what is happening without reference to the huge amount of dollars involved and where they come from and where they go. The United States spends more money for health care than any other country in the world, $180 billion a year, over $700 for each citizen. Health costs have risen dramatically, accounting for 3.5 percent of the GNP in 1929, 4.6 percent in 1950, and now almost 10 percent.

Where does all the money come from? Despite the fact that health-care expenses are the largest single reason for declarations of personal bankruptcy, fewer and fewer people are solely responsible for their own medical bills. Eighty-nine percent of the civilian noninstitutionalized population has some form of health-care coverage, however variable it may be, with 75 percent of the population covered at least in part by a nongovernmental insurance plan.

Nonetheless, the government's share of health-care expenditures has been growing relentlessly. In the early 1960s, government accounted for about one-quarter of each health-care dollar spent; now the figure is creeping up to one-half. Health expenditures have been the fastest growing component of the federal budget, and the vast majority of the increase is directly related to the introduction of Medicare and Medicaid in 1966, and the subsequent extension of Medicare coverage in 1974 to disabled persons and persons with chronic kidney disease. Three-fourths of the federal health budget is spent by the Department of Health, Education and Welfare, again principally for Medicare and Medicaid. The Veterans Administration and the Department of Defense each spend another 10 percent. No matter how many dollars the government plans to spend, it always ends up spending more. Benefit payments and administrative costs consistently exceed budgeted allocations.

Where do all these dollars go? The largest single component goes for hospital care. For Medicare patients, hospital and post-hospital care account for over two-thirds of the payments. Physicians account for a decreasing share of the health-care dollar (18.9 percent in 1976 as opposed to 21.1 percent in 1966), but many economists consider most costs to be physician-generated, under the assumption that patients go into hospitals and clinics, fill prescriptions, and get glasses and various appliances solely because doctors tell them to do so. But costs are also up because of the expensive and sophisticated technology for which American medicine has become famous, and because historically underpaid nonphysician health workers have increasingly become unionized and have demanded better salaries. Medical care remains a labor-intensive industry, and costs increase when wage increases exceed increases in productivity.

However, the single most important reason for the rise in costs has been the rise in demand. Citizens now seek care from physicians twice as often as they did fifty years ago, and they are three times as likely to be admitted to a hospital. Though the medical profession as a whole is criticized for ordering unnecessary tests and providing unnecessary services, the individual doctor facing the individual patient is far more likely to be criticized for *not* ordering tests and *not* providing services. People as patients want everything to which they feel entitled and, if in doubt, would rather have an unneeded laboratory test or X-ray than risk missing out on something which might conceivably have been useful—*especially* now that so many have been removed from any responsibility to pay. Although people are angry that health-care costs have risen so dramatically, at a personal level they have been increasingly isolated from the costs of their own care. And despite an awareness of mushrooming health costs, doctors continue to add to the expensive services, propelled by patient demands and fearful of being faulted for doing less than elusive community standards might require.

A 1976 survey of Texas physicians, for example, showed that 67 percent were ordering more X-rays than before malpractice erupted as a major concern, 66 percent were ordering more laboratory tests, and 65 percent were advising patients to obtain second opinions from other physicians. Blue Shield of California has estimated that the direct and indirect costs of "defensive medicine" add $20 billion to the nation's health-care costs each year.

The end result of the massive infusion of federal money and the voracious demand of the public for services, as well as other factors, has been an extraordinary spiraling of virtually uncontrollable health costs. Given the track record of the federal government with Medicare and Medicaid, it's hard to believe that things are likely to improve in the slightest with national health insurance.

This dramatic health-care industry growth has proliferated without any design or clear sense of purpose. Like some malignant bramble thicket, the system has spread relentlessly, without consistent rationale and without retardants, to the limit of the dollars available. Sometimes it doesn't even seem to make sense to talk about a health-care system—the word *system* implying a coherent, self-contained, efficiently operating production organization—when services are so variable, policy evolves piecemeal, cost control seems impossible, and integration of diverse and complex parts remains an elusive fantasy.

The principal problem is that there has been no consensus—or even a popular stream of opinion—defining what reasonably can be subsumed under the headings "health" or "health care." Our definitions are spongelike, reflecting a pervasive uncertainty about values, a conflict of personal desires and convenience on the one hand, and a heritage of public benevolence and a commitment to equal definitions for all, on the other.

What really is health and what really is health care?

When the World Health Organization tried to define health several years ago, it was able to do so only in relation to the absence of disease. In such circumstances, a person could be called healthy only if the doctor were unable to apply a diagnosis, which is unlikely now that the proliferation of diagnostic categories—from mild obesity to fallen arches to deviated nasal septum or myopia—makes it virtually impossible to say that any person on earth is in perfect health. A definition of such scope clearly medicalizes all of health, and adds to the general suspicion that professionals define terms for their own self-aggrandizement.

Yet the public has likewise been self-serving, if behavior can be interpreted as evidence of how people implement personal definitions. The Great Equation, as Aaron Wildavsky calls it, is that health equals medical care. When the average citizen has a health problem, he or she is far more likely to consult a doctor to be "fixed" than to attend to matters of life style and personal habits, physical environment and social conditions—over which the doctor has little or no control.

At a practical level, health as a concept is too diffuse for the average citizen to cope with, so there has been a tendency to replace the abstract and unattainable with more immediate and palpable contacts with a physician; there always seems to be something the physician can do to us, or for us, when we feel unable to do anything for ourselves. Poll after poll tells us that most people like their physicians, even as they have a growing distaste for the health professions generally; and most people like their physicians to do things for them and spend time with them, even as they are less and less willing to pay the health-care system to provide such services for others.

Because *health care* is such an unmanageable term, determining how to distribute it has likewise eluded precise organization, and decisions have often been made on a political basis, at the behest of powerful factions. In the past, the patient's ability to pay determined how much health care he or she would get, and perhaps few cared if the rich wasted their dollars on care that less financially able persons managed to do without. Conscientious physicians tried to spread their services to the needy indigent with a sliding fee scale and with idiosyncratic personal philanthropy.

Now philanthropy has been institutionalized and fee scales have been widely regulated, yet—save for extreme situations—no one knows how to define *need* for health care or to decide who should be the judge of it. Needs blend with the desires of both the giver and the receiver. The patient wants everything that might be available to anyone else and to which he or she feels entitled; and the doctor, for his or her own reasons, orders and prescribes with a free hand. Hospitals provide the best available facilities and care because they are paid to do so and can only remain competitive by keeping up with their peer institutions; and insurance companies pay the fees because they receive the dollars in premiums. Premiums are paid because they are hidden in payroll deductions or negotiated in collective bargaining agreements and workers are fearful that if their insurance policy isn't the "best," they will be deprived of their fair share of treatment. Our notions of equality, entitlement, and health blur together.

Eighty percent of those who visit the doctor come for reassurance and caring, the pollsters tell us, and most physicians who enjoy the healer role feel that providing support and caring—when we have the time and emotional energy to do it—is an important and gratifying part of our function. But at these prices, how much caring and reassurance are enough? And if indeed we are supplying more than we collectively can afford, how do we limit what we give and still perceive ourselves—and have our patients perceive us—as compassionate doctors?

While it is fascinating to talk about the problem in the abstract, this level of discourse fails to convey the immediacy of the challenge faced by the clinician. Take the Abbott family as an example. Randall Abbott is a thirty-seven-year-old sheet-metal worker who has intermittent knee pains, which have bothered him since his high-school basketball days, and intermittent low back pain; both conditions tend to act up when he is under stress. He is a hard if unenthusiastic worker, a loyal friend, a fair provider, and an inveterate dreamer who fantasizes about moving to Saudi Arabia, making big bucks, and retiring to a small farm in Idaho. He loves his wife and daughter, tries hard to tolerate his son, but hates his own parents. He enjoys his weekends and vacations and has a tendency to eat, smoke, and drink too much, and to exercise too little. All he wants from me as his physician are frequent prescriptions for pain pills, regular referrals for physical therapy, and a reasonably free hand with excuse slips which will allow him to use up every day of sick leave provided for in his union contract. He comes to the doctor once every two or three months.

However, Maria Abbott, who is thirty-four years of age, has had so much contact with doctors that her chart is thicker than a good-sized metropolitan phonebook. She has numerous physical complaints, all of which seem to be quite real to her, yet few of which can be attributed to any obvious disease processes. She takes lots of over-the-counter medicines, requests many X-rays and laboratory tests, and assumes that she will need several more operations in the next five years, though precisely for what is not clear. She has already given freely of her appendix, uterus, and gall bladder to the surgeon's knife. Her only complaint about her husband is that he snores after sex, a term which, as she uses it, means their semiregular Saturday night intercourse and his nightly masturbation. What she wants from her doctors is regular reassurance that she is performing adequately, even courageously, despite the burdens of a diseased body. Living with suffering has given her life a special flair, and she wants doctors to attest to all concerned—her extended family, her neighbors, her employer at the bakery—that her body is indeed flawed, the impediment that is to be blamed if she fails to achieve success at something she attempts.

Randall and Maria's sixteen-year-old daughter, Celia, has an appealing and zesty social manner, especially with men, but—according to her mother—is lazy, sloppy, and sarcastic at home. She takes birth-control pills, has already had one therapeutic abortion, and regularly gets "wasted" on weekends and occasional weekdays, primarily with Tequila and marijuana, but also with uppers and downers. She bites her nails a lot, has a nervous stomach, is chronically constipated, and has used enemas regularly since early childhood. She comes to the doctor whenever her mother drags her there, which is usually once every four to six weeks.

Celia's brother Roger, who is nine years old, comes in primarily for minor trauma from skateboard or bicycle injuries: puncture wounds, lacerations, bruises, scrapes, an occasional broken finger or arm. He is a bright, superficially cheerful youngster who wets his bed every now and then, for which he has been placed on medication, which seems to help "a little." He cries a lot when stressed, which drives his father up the wall but results in his mother kissing and hugging him to such an extent that doing a physical exam on Roger after one of his periodic accidents requires that I work over Maria's embracing arms and practically touch foreheads with her as I try to look in the youngster's ear.

How I as a clinician proceed with the Abbotts depends upon how I see my task with them. I have no doubt that Maria would willingly consume as much time as any group of health-care workers could give her, with the absolute conviction that truly competent medicine could take care of all her diverse needs and make her "well." If we assumed unlimited time and unlimited dollars, a group of doctors could spend major portions of their time X-raying Randall's back and knee with each resurgence of complaints, and counseling him regarding work, habitual excesses, alternative sexual behavior, and family interactions. The whole family would require at least ten hours of services a week if we seriously undertook to evaluate and treat everything related to their health: their orthopedic, surgical, pediatric, family counseling, neurological, psychiatric, obstetrical, dietary, internal medicine, gastroenterological, and emergency treatment needs stretch as far into the future as I can see.

Yet I'm not convinced that providing all of those services—as opposed to only a few of them—will make a substantial impact on their longevity or the aggregate satisfaction they get from their lives. I know we help them in some respects. I'm not totally nihilistic. I think Celia's birth control makes a difference, I hope for the better. I was pleased at how well Roger's broken arm progressed after I set it. Over the several times that I've seen Roger and his mother together, I've tried to help him become more self-sufficient in what I hope is a useful manner. "Mother," I say to the clinging Maria, "you have to let him take responsibility for his own body. If he's not able to take responsibility for that, he won't be able to take responsibility for anything, and he'll grow up to be an irresponsible adult."

I say what I do because it makes sense to me and because I can hardly refrain, given the blatant behavior before me, yet I have to believe that the Abbotts get similar counsel in places other than the doctor's office. They must hear substantially the same thing from some of their neighbors or relatives or the teachers at school. For all that I value my own perceptions of the Abbotts' family dynamics, I can't believe that my function with them is unique or that my saying what I do will automatically change their lives. For them "seeing the doctor" is a habit, a costly one, and, I believe, an overrated one. The reassurance we physicians provide—if that indeed is what it is—may make all parties involved feel transiently better, but I'm not convinced that it has any greater usefulness.

Most of the doctors I know who see the Abbotts try to take care of their multiple physical problems and to chip away at their various intra- and interpersonal problems as well; yet there is no question that we also hold the family at arm's distance. Their "needs" are too great, and our potential for significantly satisfying those needs is too small, and there are too many other families who are similar to the Abbotts in their diffuse neediness.

What we face with them is a volume and range of problems and potential demands that are impossible to meet. Few of the problems constitute illness in the sense of anatomical pathology, but illness is no longer a necessary precondition for seeing a doctor. Virtually any concern will fit under our current broad definition of health problems.

16 TEAM CARE AND TEAM POLITICS

One popular method for dealing with problems such as those presented by the Abbotts calls for the use of large numbers of nonphysician medical personnel. Physicians are too expensive, this line of reasoning goes, not responsive enough to the human needs of patients, and not numerous enough as well. The needs of the public—whatever they are—must be satisfied with the use of more and cheaper service providers.

At the turn of the century, 50 percent of all health workers were physicians. By the 1960s, health care had become an enormous industry and physicians constituted less than 10 percent of the health-care personnel. This trend has accelerated dramatically in the last twenty years, and physicians now account for less than one in twenty-five, or 4 percent, of health workers. These numbers indicate the dramatic changes that have occurred in the relationship between physicians and those who work alongside them.

The federal government now lists 665 occupational titles in the health-services industry, and this compilation neglects all those occupations that do not require formal training or that are not unique to the health industry. Examples of health occupations include cardiopulmonary technician, community health aide, electrocardiographic technician, electroencephalographic technician, extracorporeal circulation specialist, certified orthoptist, and child health associate.

One might be tempted to regard these individuals as doctors' helpers, but such a view would be simplistic and misleading. The public tends to think of the physician as an authoritarian figure, and historically this is true; many doctors tend to think of themselves that way as well. But as a practical matter, in any complex hospital or clinical setting, few physicians can get much accomplished with an authoritarian approach. Traditional patterns of dominance have yielded to the politics of collaboration. Physician leadership is no longer taken for granted—not in individual treatment decisions and not in health policy matters. Times are changing, the health-care territory is up for grabs, and so are a lot of dollars.

New careers have grown as a response to demand, in an arena where concepts and definitions are so vague as to make practically any new skill appear relevant to the care of the patient. As the health-care morass has gotten bigger and bigger, there has been a natural attempt to make specific problems more manageable by specialization and the selective use of technology. Of course, the trend started in medicine itself—with physicians who, for example, specialized first in internal medicine, then subspecialized in gastroenterology, and then finally subsubspecialized in diseases of the liver.

All of health care now seems to be a collection of technical information and services. Although the aggregate is complicated and requires breadth of training to understand, the specific technical tasks can often be mastered with far less training. In fact, someone with relatively little, but nonetheless highly specialized, training might be expected to do his or her individual task with much greater skill than a more broadly trained physician—and presumably at less expense.

Health care has gotten too complicated to be the responsibility of isolated individuals. More and more, care is delivered through a team process. The dominant role, therefore, is that of the team leader, an administrator who is not expected to have the highly developed skills of individual team members and who may not have any in-depth knowledge of the people who, as patients, have become the team's responsibility. As a result, there is less and less need for the administrator to be a physician, let alone an excellent one, and more need for the adminsitrator to be adept at coordinating the myriad parts of a task too complex overall to be understood by any of the individuals involved.

One of the ironic consequences of the democratization of health-care professionals is that in pursuit of greater responsibility, nonphysicians say: "Let us do this aspect of the physician's job. We can do the same task for less money." But once the law allows them to perform a given function, the next step is to say: "Give us more money. Equal pay for equal work. We have almost as much training as physicians."

All medicine is affected by these incursions. In all aspects of practice, nurse practitioners are moving into areas formerly reserved for physicians; throughout the country nurses are pressing for what is termed an expanded role. Physicians' assistants are gaining increasing independence. Podiatrists and physical therapists are creeping up the legs of orthopedists. Optometrists are narrowing the field of vision of ophthalmologists. Nurse midwives and lay midwives are challenging obstetricians. Technicians play a growing role in the operating room. The holistic health movement at its farthest extreme embraces psychic healers, Indian medicine men, acupuncturists, clairvoyants, spiritualists, masseurs, and yoga teachers.

In such a setting, the case of psychiatry is particularly instructive. Psychiatry can usefully be viewed as medicine's most vulnerable flank, the branch whose turmoil portends what may be ahead for the rest of the medical profession. It is here that the use of the term *health* as a societal metaphor is most prevalent, the definitions are the vaguest, the technical demands of the work the smallest, and the territorial encroachments the greatest.

To understand what has happened in psychiatry and what is happening in medicine generally, we need to look at the profession's stock in trade: the treatment of disease. In psychiatry, the term for the treatment process is *psychotherapy*. At its narrowest extreme, psychoanalytic psychotherapy, it has been defined in terms of a highly stylized interaction between a patient lying on a couch and a therapist sitting in a chair, each of whom conforms to rigorous criteria. At the other extreme is a tendency to label any help-dispensing behavior as psychotherapy, especially if the person giving the help expects to be paid for his or her time. In between is the counseling intended to be helpful—or therapeutic—which a health professional provides for a patient or client. Ultimately, the term has so many shades of meaning in today's marketplace that—without further qualification—it means nothing specific at all.

Rigorous attempts to evaluate psychotherapy began in the early 1950s and have multiplied many times over since then. The result has been an outpouring of hundreds, perhaps thousands, of papers, mostly written by individuals who want desperately to show that the practice of psychotherapy makes some difference.

The accumulated mass of data and words has been, and will continue to be, subject to conflicting interpretations, most of which can be lumped artificially and inelegantly into three camps: (1) there is no preponderance of credible evidence documenting psychotherapy's unique effectiveness; (2) the more precisely you define the patient's problem and the more precisely you define therapy, the more the evidence supports the value of certain kinds of psychotherapy in certain kinds of restricted situations; and (3) no matter how you define psychotherapy and its practitioners, a helping relationship with a therapist is likely to be beneficial to a client or a patient. Suffice it to say that no one of the camps has achieved obvious ascendancy, but their arguments produce an insistent uneasiness throughout the profession.

If accurate measurement of psychotherapy's effectiveness depends upon matching specific treatments to specific maladies, the way in which the maladies are defined and labeled makes an important difference. In psychiatry as in the rest of medicine, these labels are called diagnoses; and for a diagnosis to conform to professional standards, it must be consistent with the criteria established in the reference book *The Diagnostic and Statistical Manual of Mental Disorders* (DSM). Most lay persons tend to think of diagnoses as manifestations of natural law, accurate depictions of specific and immutable disease states. It is more correct to consider diagnoses (as they reside in the official nomenclature) as a reflection of how some people see some conditions, which they regard as diseases. There are no specific universally meaningful criteria of what constitutes mental disease, or even disease in general. Whether any individual's views prevail tends to depend upon how persuasively and persistently they are presented and whether anyone else seeks to take an opposing position and, if so, how energetically. Official diagnoses don't appear magically like condensation from unseen vapors; rather they are negotiated on a national level. The parties to the negotiations are persons who care enough about the process to take the time and energy to participate in it, often traveling across the continent to do so. Most are well intentioned, trying to sort conventional wisdom from often impassioned and competing points of view. Although most are so-called experts, their expertise may not always be an advantage. Few experts whose reputations have been established by work in a specific area want their favorite diagnoses modified in such a way as to undercut the continuing usefulness of the work they have contributed in the past. The tendency therefore has been to add diagnoses over time. In 1952 when the first *DSM* was published, it contained three major diagnostic groupings, only one of which was broken down into a significant number of subcategories. In a revision published in 1968, there were ten major categories, with a total of over two hundred official diagnoses. The current version contains twenty major categories, with considerably more diagnoses than the previous version.

For perspective, it's useful to understand that the entire process of negotiating the official psychiatric nomenclature is carried out under the auspices of the American Psychiatric Association, the national organization composed of approximately twenty-five thousand psychiatrists. Under the circumstances, it's not surprising that psychiatrists have been accused of evolving a nomenclature heavily biased by self-interest. The *DSM* is a subset of the *International Classification of Diseases,* wherein resides the standard medical nomenclature: the words and phrases used to describe the diseases, conditions, or simple variations from the norm, which may or may not cause suffering in any given individual. Ipso facto, mental disorders are medical disorders, implying that one needs to be medically trained in order to treat them.

Psychologists, not being medically trained, find this implication untenable. Why call delinquency or dependency on cigarettes a medical disorder? they ask. They are human and social disorders and we can treat them as well as you can. We'll let you call conditions like these health problems, but we won't let you call them medical problems. Ultimately, the issue may have to be decided in a court of law, with the most important arguments focusing on restraint of trade. There should be a better way to settle conceptual ambiguity than by resorting to suits between rival guilds, but no one seems to have found it yet. No one trusts closeted wisemen to make judgments on thorny conceptual issues any more. Who even believes in wisemen at this point? Instead, the tendency is to want to get issues out in the open in a court of law, where assumptions of expertise crumble as adversaries demolish one another's arguments.

The psychologists perceive, I think correctly, that in contesting psychiatry's definitions of what constitutes health and disease, they are likely to diminish psychiatry's monopolistic hold on the market and gain territorial advantages for their own profession. This is not a tactic much used by other professions against medicine, though midwives contend that pregnancy is not a disease and is therefore a suitable focus for efforts by nonphysicians.

A far more prevalent approach used by new and expanding professions has been to focus not on basic concepts and definitions but rather on economic privileges, utilizing political clout and access to legislators as the vehicle to success. Its principal ploy has been the development of longer and more technically oriented professionalized education, offering more prestigious credentials. The key element in the success of this approach has been the fact that many legislators see territorial expansion by certain groups as meeting the genuine needs and desires of their constituents. Again, the case of psychiatry is instructive.

An event that occurred while I was a member of the American Psychiatric Association Committee on Psychiatric Nursing is particularly illustrative. The APA committee was one of those harmless anachronisms to be found in any organizational structure. It had been started some time in the past, probably for a good reason, but had persisted far beyond its usefulness because no one wanted to go to the trouble of disbanding it. We committee members were flown twice yearly to Washington, D.C., from our far-flung home bases, and thus enjoyed the illusion of participating in organizational politics at no expense to ourselves.

On this particular day, I had been a member of the committee for a year and a half, and was already familiar with the format of the meetings. Mostly we chatted in a sociable and directionless fashion, thinking about ways in which our group could foster mutually amicable relationships between psychiatrists and psychiatric nurses. Nothing of much consequence was ever decided, but neither did we generate any unpleasantness. It was a fine, civilized gathering, and when the meeting was concluded we would adjourn for cocktails and the continued satisfaction of one another's company.

Though the avowed purpose was to promote goodwill and inter-professional alliances with nurses, the tone of the meetings was more paternalistic than cooperative. "How can we help *them?*" we wondered. What could we doctors do to help nurses get better working conditions and more recognition? While all of us had received ample assistance from psychiatric nurses in clinical situations back home, there was never any thought that nurses might have anything to contribute to us nationally, at a political level, much less that they might pose a threat to our professional hegemony. Everyone knew that doctors called the shots when it came to making policy—at least we thought we did.

In September of 1975, a liaison representative of the American Nursing Association, a likeable and spirited woman, joined our meeting. She had come because she wanted to request APA support of a bill pending in Congress; and, in her engagingly articulate way, she went on to describe in detail what was involved.

The Inouye Bill, sponsored by the senator from Hawaii, was designed to promote independent functioning by psychiatric nurses. Everyone nodded. That was okay. Many psychiatric nurses were capable of greater autonomy than the law currently allowed. As a matter of fact, the ANA representative went on, the bill called for qualified psychiatric nurses to have hospital privileges similar to those of psychiatrists.

Alarm spread through the room. Nurses admit and discharge their own patients? Write orders in the chart? Perhaps prescribe medications? Have full voting privileges on hospital staffs? No, we really couldn't support that.

But she wasn't through. The bill further required that hospitals refusing to provide psychiatric nurses with hospital privileges on an equal footing with psychiatrists be denied all federal health insurance payments such as those derived from Medicare and Medicaid.

"My God," somebody said aloud. "Over fifty percent of fees at my hospital come from those sources." Others reacted with similar astonishment and vigorous protest. The discussion went on for some time, with the consternation of the committee members abundantly clear. There was a presumption built into this bill that was profoundly upsetting.

The worst was yet to come.

After everyone had had a chance to comment, and the comments themselves were becoming repetitious, the ANA speaker again asserted herself. "Gentlemen and lady," she said, with a nod to the one female psychiatrist in the room, "I won't take up your time any longer. We would like your support and, failing that, we would prefer not to have your opposition. But I didn't come here to beg. There are well over a million nurses in this country, and only twenty-five thousand psychiatrists. Congress and its constituency are receptive to the notion of expanding roles for nonphysician health personnel. This bill may not pass this year, but eventually one like it will pass. The flow of history is with us."

And of course she is correct.

The report of the President's Commission on Mental Health, released in 1978, recommends that "the consumer should have a choice of provider and provider systems." The carefully phrased statement may be interpreted to mean that physicians should no longer consider themselves to have a monopolistic hold on the market. The commission goes on to say that "all covered services must be rendered by, or under the direct clinical supervision of, a physician, psychologist, social worker, or nurse with earned doctorate or master's degree."

Psychologists, now well over fifty thousand strong, not only outnumber psychiatrists by about two to one, but, as we have seen, are effectively challenging heretofore sacrosanct physician prerogatives. Psychologists are now licensed or certified in almost all of the fifty states and therefore are legally able to provide services independently of physician supervision, and to bill third-party insurers, also often without physician supervision. As their numbers increase, psychologists' political leverage will inevitably increase too, and psychology is experiencing a dramatic mushrooming of growth. Estimates suggest that there are five thousand new Ph.D.'s in psychology each year from a pool of over twelve thousand first-year psychology graduate students, compared to several hundred new psychiatrists each year.

One hundred thousand persons have master's degrees in social work in this country, and an evolutionary expansionism similar to that of nursing has been occurring in the social-work profession. Many lay persons tend to think of social workers as caseworkers employed within a service agency, but clinical psychotherapy practice—though up to now somewhat restricted by legislation—has traditionally been the most prestigious activity for social-work practitioners. Barriers that restrict social workers from competing effectively with psychiatrists are crumbling. In 1976 the California legislature passed AB2374, putting social workers on a financial par with psychiatrists in all outpatient care funded by private insurance programs operating in the state. The only requirement was that the therapy be undertaken at the recommendation of a licensed physician, who need not be a psychiatrist.

Major established professions are not the only ones eating into the territory. In February 1978 the Board of Regents of the University of California approved a new program leading to a doctorate in mental health (DMH). The nonmedical curriculum was designed to produce students who would be better clinicians than psychologists and better theoreticians than psychiatrists. Though no licensing yet exists for these graduates, the program's sponsors are seeking a new licensing category, which will allow limited prescribing privileges restricted to so-called psychoactive agents—essentially tranquilizers and related drugs.

Marriage and family counselors now have a national certifying organization, The American Association of Marriage and Family Counselors, requiring training at a master's degree level, and have already obtained licensing of practitioners in many states. While practitioners call themselves counselors, the national organization's official brochure mentions supervised clinical work only in the areas of "individual therapy, marital therapy, and family therapy." Despite the organization's name, counseling is nowhere mentioned. The implication is clear: counseling is the same as psychotherapy, and we can do it.

The American Association of Sex Educators, Counselors, and Therapists certifies therapists who hold at least a master's degree, and the field is growing rapidly. Twenty-five programs now offer doctorate degrees in rehabilitation counseling, the majority of whose graduates work with the mentally ill. Music therapy aims at "the restoration, maintenance, and improvement of mental and physical health," and by 1978, fifty-seven universities and colleges were offering baccalaureate degrees in the field; several are beginning to offer master's degrees. Nine major universities grant master's degrees in art therapy. Some call it art psychotherapy and use the process to "assist in the understanding and working through of emotional problems." Dance therapy is described by its practitioners as "psychotherapeutic use of movement as a process which furthers the emotional and physical integration of the individual." Dance therapists currently must have a bachelor's degree, but the profession is in the process of being upgraded. By 1983, therapists will be required to have a master's degree.

Occupational therapy began as a profession when somebody noticed that psychiatric patients who were busy recovered more quickly than those who weren't. Now there are over forty college programs turning out occupational therapists with bachelor's degrees, and perhaps twenty preparing students at the master's level.

In 1965 the first two-year college program for mental-health workers was begun in an extension program at Purdue University. There are now over a hundred and forty such programs, which seek to prepare mental-health generalists rather than assistants to any of the existing mental-health professions. If they aren't to be our assistants, do they consider themselves to be our peers? Can they practice independently?

Persons who, in a previous era, were called attendants in the state hospital have gradually upgraded their role. With time, their title became psychiatric technician or mental-health technician, and they sought first certification and then licensure. As they developed professional standards and professional standing, they formed a national organization—the National Association of Human Services Technologists. Their requirements are steadily rising from the present minimum of a high-school education and one year of specialized training to an emerging standard of a certificate from a two-year college or an associated arts degree leading to licensure.

My point in reciting all this is to convey some sense of the vast numbers of people with increasingly lengthy training who are converging on the patient in the name of helping. At what time will all of us helpers become so numerous and so thoroughly trained that we spend more time stumbling over one another than actually helping our patients? At what time will each person's relative contribution seem so trivial that the extensive training will no longer seem worthwhile? With so many people looking after one or another fragment of patient care, it is likely that before very long no one will feel any identification with the supposed end product of his or her work: the overall health of the patient.

Yet it is precisely that person, the citizen-patient-consumer who— via demands for increased amounts of ill-defined services—makes all this professional and paraprofessional overgrowth not only possible, but apparently necessary. And as the demands increase, as they show every appearance of doing, the situation can only get worse.

These demands take many forms, but at the level of health legislation, most prominent are those of various special-interest consumer and provider groups, each claiming to speak for the health and welfare of the "little person" with a clarity of vision that no one else has. Everybody wants something, and the language for achieving those somethings is explicit. Each demand for each special-interest group claims to enhance accessibility of services, improve manpower utilization, develop structural change, set quality-control standards, and monitor cost effectiveness. And each demand, seemingly so sensible in itself, mires the system in a confusing morass of greater cost and complexity, without any internal logic.

The 1960s and 1970s—the latter called by some the decade of the consumer—focused on the rights of the average citizen confronting insensitive monolithic institutions, from General Motors to meat packers to banks. In the early 1960s, these rights were codified into a Consumers' Bill of Rights, which reflects a deep mistrust among consumers that has been generated by countless examples of avarice, carelessness, and duplicity among producers of all kinds of goods and services. And nowhere has this mistrust been more bitter and destructive than in medical care, where the patient-consumer feels especially vulnerable and where the services are intensely personal, sometimes carrying life-and-death implications.

Go into any major medical center and watch the admissions procedure as a patient enters the hospital. More and more often, the process is so structured as to resemble the reading of the Miranda rights by police officers to apprehended persons. The patient is warned of rights, not only to make certain that he or she knows them (which often is already true), but also to emphasize that the physician and hospital know them as well: "You have a right to know all information relevant to your care, to ask questions and to question the answers, to be informed about the nature and purpose of procedures, the risks, the cost, the likely outcome, as well as the available alternatives to the procedures recommended. Most of all you have the right to refuse anything—including diagnostic as well as therapeutic procedures, and of course hospitalization itself." The fact that this indoctrination has taken place must then be documented by duly witnessed signatures on a standard form which attests to the continuing wariness of both doctor and patient, the symbol of distrust between them.

Daniel Bell has said that the conflict between the professional and the consumer is the post-industrial service sector's equivalent of the industrial era's conflict between capitalist and labor. Whatever the formulation, there is no question that more and more physicians feel mistrusted and resented, insufficiently appreciated, too often at odds with their patients, at a state of personal and professional crisis—in a word, besieged.

They are assaulted from within by the impossibility of knowing everything they feel they have to know, and of providing persistently skilled care in the Hippocratic tradition to all those who seem so diffusely, sometimes maddeningly, needy. They are assaulted from without by a system that removes authority and forces adherence to conflicting allegiances, by a patient-public that increasingly assumes an adversary stance, and by a society that devalues and sometimes even seems to punish experience, expertise, and the assumption of responsibility.

Complaints about medicine in general—and psychiatry in particular—bombard the physician at every turn. The criticisms cover the entire range of our activities. We provide overcare for the healthy and wealthy few and neglect the suffering multitudes. We don't do much for the aged, the retarded, the minorities, or the disadvantaged—and we do a terrible job when we try. We don't accomplish anything with the violent, except ineptly or even maliciously locking up the harmless under the guise of treating the dangerous. We are too often profiteers, who are frequently incompetent and who don't keep up with the latest developments unless we're forced to. We have used diagnoses in an idiosyncratic manner, sloppily covering our social judgments with pseudoscientific labels, stigmatizing our patients with semantic stupidity. Our fuzzy science isn't scientific enough, and our awkward art is not artful enough. We are peculiar as individuals, perhaps even crazier than our craziest patients. We are eager to trample on other people's rights if it suits our purpose, and we try to control our co-workers as well as our patients—and all for selfish purposes. In the courtroom we are prostitutes who will testify to anything if the pay is enough, thereby revealing that our expertise is so subjective as to be a sham. At one extreme, we are oppressive and totalitarian, conscious instruments of political control. At the other, we are dupes who compound misery by describing it in terms of individual defect and disease, thereby mitigating against more sensible and more political definitions and solutions. Ivan Illich says that the medical establishment, we doctors, have ourselves become a threat to health.

Buffoons and incompetents and crooks have attracted enormous media attention and shape the public's changing view of the entire profession. The surgical-equipment salesman lacking a high-school diploma comes into the operating room to bail out befuddled orthopedic surgeons, and then talks grinningly of his exploits on TV. A prominent psychiatrist is convicted of having sexual relations with his patient in the name of therapy, and the whole seamy episode, in addition to getting enormous media attention at the time, becomes the subject of a movie and a book entitled *Betrayal*. Medicine has been buffeted and reshaped by malpractice suits, and all in public view. Physicians have been charged with fraud, the bilking of insurance companies, and the mismanagement of public funds. The profession has been depicted as an inbred, smarmy brotherhood, selfishly standing in the way of national health insurance and keeping out women and minorities. Doctors refuse to testify against one another and hide homicidal mistakes as if the loss of life were an incidental event in a professional game.

Medicine and psychiatry as professions have followed a recognizable sequence: first suspect, then fashionable, then familiar, and now increasingly superfluous. In some ways, the sequence is an inevitable consequence of psychiatry's greatest contribution: teaching all of us to look beneath the surface of people and events. In the process, selfless servants were seen as other than selfless—and heroic leaders and authorities were seen as other than heroic. Psychiatry has made it more difficult for us to sustain the belief in our own illusions, and has made us feel naïve for depending on an authority based primarily on tradition. All our institutions have taken a tumble, but perhaps psychiatry and medicine most of all.

The physicians of today, raised with the ideals of the past, often find it difficult to function comfortably in the evolving system of the present. Their internal demands are in conflict with external realities. The real world in which they function fails to support the inner sense of dedication which many doctors feel, and which the public seems to want doctors to feel: to be special to the patient, and to make the relationship between doctor and patient personal and uniquely powerful. The failure of expectations has practical consequences too; for without this specialness, the doctor's power to influence and to heal is weakened.

For more and more of these physicians, to try to exist in both worlds—to be a team player in addition to carrying ultimate legal responsibility for the patient, and feeling ultimate moral responsibility—becomes too much. Doctors lack confidence and a professional sense of purpose. How can we struggle with life-and-death issues, with the ethical problems of daily practice, when we are no longer confident that we are worthy of such an honor and responsibility? Confused and dispirited by the vague and conflicting definitions and demands around us, we question our own self-definition and doubt the intelligence of the demands we have traditionally placed upon ourselves.

We feel overburdened and depleted. Burned out. Demand exceeds resources, and there is nothing left, save a glimmer of hope that the future will be better.

National health insurance is in the wings, as it has been for the past three decades and more, growing in size and potential impact. When it comes, it will determine the fabric of this country's health care, creating a nationwide, standardized pattern that will have an impact on individual citizens as great as that of the postal system or the internal revenue system. Once it's here, it will be no easier to change than either of those vast governmental institutions.

As doctors, my colleagues and I wonder what these developments will mean for our profession. What will they mean for me? What will my relationships with patients be like in another score of years? Will times be easier or more difficult?

Now I think I know. I can see what is ahead, and—from a selfish point of view—I don't like it.

17 A PROGNOSIS FOR THE DOCTOR-PATIENT RELATIONSHIP

The next several decades are going to be brutalizing for conscientious physicians who wish to be complete physicians to patients they want to see as whole human beings, who try to do it all.

Highly technical scientific medicine will be regarded as a commodity, the theoretic universal availability of which will be limited by bureaucrats whose primary task will be cost control. Issues of accountability will be justified in terms of assuring quality, but with the tacit understanding to limit services. The easiest method will simply be to keep people waiting in line until they find it preferable to do without rather than to continue waiting in line. Sins of omission in medical care will be preferred to sins of commission, just because they tend to be cheaper. In an era where inflation and recession are dominant realities, and with national health insurance imminent, we have no other choice.

Given these requirements, the profession as a whole will define its task and its methods by borrowing the concepts—if not the language—of industrialization. Just as no single worker can economically build a car in the Ford motor plant, no doctor will be able to take full responsibility for all aspects of a human being's health care. Those who try will be found wanting when measured by uniform standards related to production, efficiency, and uniformity.

Despite all the rhetoric to the contrary, physicians will continue in the direction of further specialization, to facilitate the partial-task orientation of the production line as opposed to the whole-task orientation of the craftsman. The economy of rapid processing will squeeze out the artistry and humanism in the care of patients. No one will have the time and energy and guts to buck the trend. Technology and bureaucratic services will use up all the health-care dollars and all the human energy.

Diseases will be defined more and more precisely in order to fit the process of health care into the production-line model. Doctors will not be allowed to treat whole patients because whole human beings elude precise definition and you can't measure the cost effectiveness of treatment at such a murky level.

If a peptic ulcer is to be redefined in any way, it will have to be as a duodenal ulcer or esophageal ulcer; the qualifying terms must be anatomical or physiological, objective and precise, because that is all the system can tolerate and afford. There will be no room to describe the ulcer in more human terms: for example, as the personal response of a black police officer who works in a racially turbulent precinct and who is simultaneously struggling with divorce and the death of a parent. That information, having no relevance to the production line, will simply be a distraction and will have to be selectively ignored.

Psychological and social services will have no place in the structure, or they will be foisted onto the least credentialed and least experienced workers in the health-care system—if only to keep costs down.

The doctor, as the most highly trained health-care worker and therefore the most expensive, will be confined increasingly to the most technical and specialized tasks on the one hand, and to cost-limiting positions guarding access to expensive resources on the other. The physician will stand at key spots in health-care funnels and operate the stopcocks which limit flow. Access to expensive services—such as specialized hospitalizations, rarefied diagnostics, complicated procedures, and disability judgments—will be allocated by persons with the most highly specialized and subspecialized credentials. The ostensible and partially honest rationale will concern quality of care ("This stuff is too technical for anyone but the most highly trained to understand and use competently"), but the function served by the system will be to limit costs.

Increasingly, the doctor will be perceived by patients as someone aloof, interested solely in disease and the choreography of treatment, often standing in the way of what the patient perceives as entitlements, out of touch with the patient as a human being.

The greatest clashes between doctor and patient will come when the two are dealing with hard-to-define clinical problems, in institutional settings with highly developed cost consciousness, where the patients' expectations conflict with bureaucratic guidelines to which the doctor is required to adhere. No matter how hard the conscientious doctor tries to make things otherwise, the patient's perception of impersonality of care will seem uncomfortably accurate, initially and especially in metropolitan health-care institutions, but gradually elsewhere as well.

Patients will not be satisfied with such a trend—as indeed they are not now—and will demand that a more human dimension be a part of medical care. In their growing sophistication, they will understand that there is more to healing than technical procedures, and they will understand the value of human relationships in fostering healing. They will hunger for personal care, as their doctors persist in treating disease impersonally. They will be frustrated and angry at the disparity between what they seek and what they receive, and many will fail to accept straightforward explanations of their doctors' limitations. They will seek to replace their apparently callous physicians, whose behavior is so vexing and inexplicable, with warm human beings who seem really to care about the human dimension. As the public berates the veterinary tendency of modern medicine, the number and variety of nonphysician health-care workers will continue to rise in an attempt to fill this compassion gap.

The arrival of all these people in the health-care arena will put still more pressure on the physician to become superspecialized—in part because physicians will cherish the sophisticated knowledge that elevates them above the crowd and helps them feel unique amid the mass of health-care workers, and in part because these less highly trained persons can perform the less technical jobs with adequate skill at lower cost. Those with lesser credentials will have another advantage: they will be held to lower standards of accountability and punished less severely for their lapses in performance. Treatment of the whole human being will gradually be taken away from the physician.

All physicians will feel the pressures: surgeons, internists, psychiatrists. Specialists in psychiatry will find themselves retreating to smaller and smaller areas, in which their medical training allows them to retain a certain measure of hegemony. Psychiatry will narrow its scope to the kinds of mental illness that can be defined in biological terms, and will look harder and harder for a biological component in any variation in individual psychic performance.

Even family practice, and even its most holistically oriented practitioners, will be nudged along the same pathway. Ninety percent of the problems that come into the general physician's office can be handled effectively by someone less highly trained, and as those persons—nurse practitioners, physicians' assistants, health technicians of various sorts—become more available, the tendency will be for physicians to act in a supervisory role, having less instead of more to do with individual patients, unless the patients are actually sick enough and their disorders complicated enough to demand a higher level of technical skill. More and more, the family practitioner's job will be to focus on such technical procedures, sign forms and prescriptions, and take administrative responsibility for the actions of others.

Matters related to wellness and health—as opposed to illness—may remain complicated at a conceptual level but not at a practical level. Once principles of "healthy living" are established and documented, they tend to be readily comprehensible by the many rather than by the few. Health counseling will therefore be the function of nonphysician health workers, who will call in physicians only when technical advice is necessary. Physicians will be seen as too highly trained and too expensive to concern themselves with wellness; their job will continue to be treating disease, most particularly that small aspect of it which is beyond the competence of other health professionals.

Physicians have been widely denounced for the high level of their incomes, and probably appropriately so. But what has been unique about physicians has not been their financial motivation—many people in our society covet large incomes and the prestige that goes with them—but, rather, the profession's success in this respect *and* the fact that it has been operating in exclusive territory, has had monopolistic license. But that license is now ceasing to be monopolistic. Nurses and pharmacists and optometrists and physicians' assistants are angling for prescribing privileges, and will be getting them (at first on a limited basis); and their growing incomes will reflect the change. Psychologists and nurses, now lobbying for admitting privileges at hospitals, will be getting them; and they will demand higher fees in recognition of their increased responsibility. Many other groups are eroding the physician's once exclusive turf, with the result that doctors no longer feel themselves unique and special except when caring for the most complicated of diseases.

Since national health insurance will never produce all the benefits expected of it, its supporters will push for more and more drastic changes in the system after it has been established. People who seek health care will feel betrayed by changes that were supposed to make things better but somehow only make them worse. People will want to punish the health-care system for its insensitivity and perceived cruelty, and its failure to meet expectations.

The people who make policy and who advise our lawmakers will be increasingly angry and frustrated—either as the recipients of unsatisfying care on the one hand, or failed clinicians on the other—and in desperation will try to mandate the way doctors and patients should behave. As a consequence, clinicians will feel even more restricted and regulated than they now do, and morale will deteriorate further.

Erosion of morale is one way of producing political change, and indeed that will be the eventual effect. Doctors will sooner or later cease their futile fighting against changes that seem inevitable, and the time will come when the profession of medicine ceases to exist as a unique entity.

What does all this mean to the average citizen—and to the average health-care worker?

For you, the citizen, it means that your search for a compassionate, technically competent personal physician whom you can call your own will increasingly be in vain. If you know such a person now—someone who gives technically skillful care, who is not burned out, who remains compassionate—treasure him or her. There are such people, a dying breed though they may be, and they need all the support and appreciation they can get to resist the pressures to become something else.

If you are already disillusioned with physicians and are placing your hopes on the new categories of health workers, your satisfaction is likely to be transitory. The "new breed" workers will probably elude the pressures which created them only so long as they are flushed with the excitement of new and challenging accomplishments, as long as they feel special and unique, and as long as the system doesn't subject them to the same impersonal standards of accountability and productivity that dominate the established professions in their established roles.

With time and the routinization of their roles, these workers will feel the same vulnerability as have others before them. Psychological care of the seriously ill and needy is emotionally draining, and these nonphysicians will feel overwhelmed. They will lack the credentials and status and priestly vestments that could set them apart and protect them from the desperation of the masses of clients. In their struggle, they themselves will seek emotional support from physicians and others in positions of administrative authority. They will be told how valuable their contribution is, how important, but they will know that the people saying the words won't mean them, and wouldn't do the same work for the same rewards. Like the physicians before them, they will tend to fall into the same gatekeeping postures, to process patients with the least pain to themselves. Many will seek to flee their sense of inadequacy and guilt by accumulating more credentials, focusing more on technical skills, and having less contact with patients, especially those whose treatment is inherently most frustrating and least fulfilling.

Patients will feel at the mercy of health-care workers, and health-care workers will feel at the mercy of patients and an insensitive and oppressive health-care system. Everyone will feel ineffectual in the clutches of a bureaucracy whose dimensions are beyond individual understanding.

Malpractice suits will become increasingly numerous and increasingly expensive, and their targets will widen: nurse practitioners, health technicians, and other health-care workers who will no longer be able to hide under the physicians' umbrella. As a consequence, health-care workers will retreat from the care of the sickest patients or those with the most challenging problems, where the probability of dire results is the greatest and malpractice risk proportionately high.

Ultimately, health care will become an array of technical services, and whatever compassion and tenderness you encounter will be incidental. When the post office clerk knows you by name, it adds a pleasant note to your day, and may in fact have resulted from your having treated the post office clerk like a human being; but it's not something that you can expect as a part of your daily experience, unless you live in one of those few towns where everyone knows everyone else anyhow.

Medical care is a part and product of the contemporary culture. Compassion and tenderness as routine features in medical care are only likely to occur in a society that fosters a nurturing environment. This is not true of our society, so these qualities will be more conspicuous by their absence than by their presence—and it makes little sense to waste much time in angry resentment that this is so.

As people come to recognize these trends, they will tend to stay away from medical care whenever possible. We will return to a shared cultural view which holds that people seek hospital care—and often outpatient medical care as well—only in the event of life-threatening circumstances.

The only people who will cling consistently to bureaucratized health care in non-life-threatening circumstances will be those who are severely disturbed or grossly impaired; and with few exceptions, they will be able to elicit caring only from persons who are paid to dispense it, in settings that diffuse the intensity of the contact.

What we will have lost most of all is that wonderful sense that when we are sickest and most needy, we will be looked after by someone whose credentials and trustworthiness and understanding and acceptance of us as unique and valuable individuals are beyond question. Instead, the responsibility for coordinating our own health care will fall on us alone; and accompanying it will be the guilt and sense of personal failure that are part of knowing that when things go wrong, we have no one to blame but ourselves.

Perhaps this is the bitterest pill of all: that if you want to be assured of compassionate tenderness when you are sick or troubled, you will have to find it among friends and relatives and people who know you. If the concern they can offer you is insufficient, it is unlikely that the health-care system will be able to make up the difference. That you even expect it to do so is a relic of a bygone age.

18 NOTES TO WOULD-BE HEALERS

If you are a conscientious health-care worker, or more particularly, a physician—someone who gives a damn, someone who views the trends I have outlined here with alarm or horror—what does all this mean for you? And who am I to advise you? I who am at once a psychiatrist and a generalist, not content to label myself solely as either one, simultaneously participant and observer, harboring gloomy forecasts for the doctor-patient relationship as I have come to understand it?

I see myself as a fairly ordinary physician, contending with my own variable motivation and skill, in less than ideal circumstances, trying to meet my patients' expectations as well as my own—and failing at the task more often than I would like. Why else write this book?

I recognize now that I came into medicine with unrealistic expectations, believing that by virtue of being a conscientious physician I would become someone who was beyond the ordinary. Not godlike or saintly as some stereotypes would have it, but special in a very human way, abundant in qualities of patience, wisdom, fairness, resourcefulness, generosity of spirit, and faithfulness to duty.

With more experience, I have learned that these qualities are not mine simply by Hippocratic inheritance. Rather I must earn them on my own, not just once but dozens of times daily. Without constant effort, they slip from my fingers, and I have found I don't have the energy to make that effort as often as I—or others—would like. There are simply too many patients and too many others with demands on my loyalty. Their expectations of me are collectively beyond my resources and too often in conflict. I feel inadequate, a feeling which comes not only as a result of my own attempts and failures, but also from watching the attempts and failures of many of my colleagues. Many of them are struggling even more painfully than I. I feel frightened watching some fall by the wayside. I understand their anguish, and I am afraid.

There are no heroes any more. People work out their own solutions now, and usually find them less than ideal. I have made my own compromises, and I commend them to no one else. They are personal and flawed, and inevitably they will change with time.

I can't accept lavishing care on the wealthy few when so many are in need, so I give smaller dollops of care to greater numbers. I work for a salary in a place that is as fair to me and my patients as any I could find. My employer offers reasonable care at reasonable prices to vast numbers of patients, and I don't have to worry about bankrupting patients with the care I give. I am grateful to have the job. It's a good job as jobs go, but still a job. It's not the hallowed calling that I once imagined, not an automatic ticket to respect and deference.

My personal resources are too limited for me to become emotionally involved with so many patients, so I give of myself sparingly and draw elaborate boundaries between my personal and professional lives. When I am with my patients, I do my damnedest to be sensitive, caring, compassionate, respectful, and technically adept, according to my judgment of their needs. But the work exhausts me. Twelve hours a day is all I can take, and not too many such days in a row either. I don't take call, and I often leave the phone off the hook when I am home. I rarely stop to give first aid at accidents, I rarely provide medical care to friends or neighbors, and I more rarely still become friends with people who are or have been my patients. My attempts to separate my professional and private lives are unending but alas inconsistent: I never identify myself as "Doctor" when making dinner or hotel reservations or try to use my medical degree for leverage in nonprofessional settings, but I'm happy that my medical degree ensures that I will always have a job and that my credit rating is almost automatically above suspicion.

I don't practice psychotherapy now in any traditional sense. I haven't got sufficient emotional reserves to do the kind of job I would like to do. The work seems to me to be too burdensome, without the cultural support that ennobles the endeavor and makes the burdens tolerable. Perhaps in the future I will feel differently. For the moment, I try to be therapeutic to my patients' psyches, while I diagnose and treat their bodies.

I accept that in working as a general practitioner and in trying to care for many patients as whole human beings, I will inevitably perform inadequately in some specific situations. I will make mistakes, and some people will die as a consequence. I rationalize that my fallibility is the curse of the generalist, and that despite this, the generalist's more global understanding helps many where the specialist's narrow focus is of little use. To compensate, I request many consultations from colleagues, and I constantly remind my patients of my ignorance and limitations, so that their own wariness will help protect them. Their health is their responsibility, I tell them, and I rigorously avoid making decisions for those among them who want the "expert" to do so.

I accept that the process of providing quality care, and the process of documenting one's ability to provide such care, are only tangentially related. To the extent that I have embraced the latter, I have done so as an inveterate gamesperson. It is an opportunity for diversion from patient care and an opportunity for competition in an arena that is ultimately meaningless but one in which I nonetheless have some skills. I fill in patients' charts in a way that will probably make medical auditors happy. When I take the inevitable shortcuts, I try to gloss over them, hiding their existence in my indecipherable handwriting. I collect CME credits and frame the certificates and place them on my walls, as evidence to support not my narcissism but my cynicism. They will be useful to point to when the inevitable happens and I am sued for malpractice. I am overdue as it is.

I accept that patient care protocols also offer me relative protection from malpractice suits if I follow them, though I don't believe the patient is necessarily better off. I try to retain my individuality separate from the protocols in silly little ways which are nonetheless important to me: idiosyncratic mannerisms and figures of speech; therapeutic nostrums that no one else prescribes, and diagnostic labels that no one else would ever use. These are like my signature—unique and personal. They reaffirm my singularity and the singularity of my relationship with each patient in an increasingly regimented medical world.

I have my greatest difficulties with matters of conflicting allegiances, and I have found no consistent guiding principle to help me choose among my patient, my employer, and various other administrative and governmental bodies when their demands are in conflict. Sometimes I enter into collusion with a patient and say, in essence: "You and I are together in a relationship which remains special and personal, and the two of us will ignore the rest." Sometimes I shrug my shoulders helplessly and say, "I know what you would like me to do, but the law or my employer requires that I behave in a different fashion. My hands are tied." Sometimes I say to hell with all of them, and take a path solely of my own choosing, rationalizing that my own demands are of equal importance to all the rest and that I must look after my own needs lest I falter as have so many of my colleagues.

The conflict of allegiances concerns not only institutions but also ideas, values, concepts, and the methods each of us relies on for everyday problem-solving. Where should I turn for reliable instruction in trying to be helpful to people who come to me for guidance? In truth, I am a creature of Western medicine, and the medical-surgical hospital is my spiritual home. I believe in scholarship and the scientific method, but in practice I operate largely on the basis of intuition and habit. I have struggled to find solid conceptual footing in Freudian and behavioral psychology, as well as in medical physiology and anatomy and pathology, and more recently in meditation and holistic health practices, but at heart I remain an American pragmatist. My most important operational question is: "How can I be most helpful to this person who is my patient?" To the extent that I have a single guiding principle in diagnosis and treatment, it is "First do no harm." More and more, I find myself relying on the passage of time to reveal all, and to heal what it will.

I try to avoid taking clinical responsibility for human problems that have come to be thought of—erroneously, I believe—as medical problems. Alcoholism, drug addiction, accident-proneness, self-destructive behavior—my profession may call them diseases, but I don't believe it for a minute. I can find satisfaction in treating people with such human problems only by defining my task in a very limited fashion, by patching them up as best I can and releasing them to go on doing the things that they find pleasant or necessary but that do much harm to their bodies and often to other people. Living wisely is an individual responsibility, and we all have to learn it for ourselves.

I look at the nonphysicians who work at my side, most of them struggling conscientiously for new levels of mastery and recognition. I teach them and encourage them and sometimes learn from them, taking vicarious pride in the attainments of each individual, yet in the aggregate I view them all with a sense of foreboding. I feel the uniqueness of my own role eroding, and I become defensive and protective of my professional prerogatives. Though I would encourage each individual to perform to capacity, I cannot be sure how I would vote on issues of expanded licensure for various nonphysician health professionals. I would like to think I would vote with my conscience, but my conscience is too variable to be predictable.

I struggle too with the issue of medicine's wealth. In the abstract, I readily concede that many physicians make too much money for the public good, yet at a personal level I would fight to retain every penny of my own salary and would of course be happy to accept a raise. I would, if necessary, work for less money, but I would prefer to work for more. Money is a prime workplace motivator in our culture, no less so for physicians than for others, including our patients.

In a pluralistic society with an economic system that is a hodgepodge of democratic socialism, meritocracy, and entrepreneurialism, what rewards are necessary to keep our healers healing? How does one define human suffering in a way which is rational, which is respectful of human sensitivities, yet which provides dignity and rewards to persons who try to be of help and who study and work to exhaustion in order to do so? How do you get good people to stay in clinical care and to function with high morale without killing themselves?

I carry on these internal discussions weekly, if not daily. Sometimes I get angry and impatient with myself for griping and obsessing. "Shut up," I say to myself, "shut up and do your job. Lots of people have it lots worse."

In an age of cynicism and self-doubt and disenchantment with the work ethic generally and with the demands of difficult work specifically, it is the fashion to disdain dedication and selflessness. Aspirations toward nobility of character are not only suspect but are mocked as foolish pretense. Both the aspirations and the mockery battle within me. I try not to let the battles intrude upon my behavior with patients. Usually I'm all right so long as I'm with the patient and focusing on the problem that brings the patient to me.

Sometimes the battle is only retrospective, a cerebral jousting with dogma and labels entirely dissociated from the imperatives I feel in a patient's presence. I saw a woman, for example, who came to the emergency room crying hysterically, barely able to walk or to speak a coherent sentence, suffering a madonna's anguish, her three teenage children the victims of a senseless, fatal auto accident. I approached her with dread—what could I possibly say? Yet in her presence, instinct and professional training and habit overcame my reticence. I held her hands in mine and talked with her, the words coming in fragments, phrases about meaninglessness and suffering, about love and bereavement, about God and the search for meaning. Gradually the hysterics dissipated and then there were only her deep diaphragmatic sobs, and the two of us sitting knee to knee, our hands clasped together. Slowly, through the tears in her eyes, she saw the watering in mine, and squeezed my hands to comfort me. Then, her composure regained, she left, her awesome dignity leaving me humble and contemplative behind her.

As I started for my next patient, a younger colleague met me in the hallway and inquired about what had transpired between the woman and me. "Did you psychotherapize her?" he asked. I nodded, numb, at a loss to know how to respond otherwise.

For many people, the term *psychotherapy* has come to be synonymous with our attempts to treat patients as people, as understandingly and humanely as we can, separate from procedures and techniques. The longer I practice, the less credence I put in the various diagnostic and therapeutic phrases that clutter a physician's professional life, and the less patience I have with bureaucratic attempts to categorize what I do. We have cloaked our skills and perspectives in such a complicated theoretic and semantic fabric that the simple beauty of one human being assisting another has been all but obscured.

With most patients I see, and in most aspects of my work, I maintain a superficial cheerfulness. It makes the day go more easily, and by now it's an established habit. Yet over the past several years, there is no question but that I have been depressed. Not morbidly, I hope, but depressed nonetheless. Much of that depression has been a consequence of the complex changes going on within my profession and the accusations that have been hurled at physicians by those whose expectations we have failed to meet. Criticism has served a useful purpose in the past and will in the future, but too often I think the level of insensitive invective makes things worse rather than better.

As a practitioner, I need to be able to assume that my colleagues and I are competent. Doctors will be more caring and giving when we aren't defensive. We need to know that we are perceived as persons of goodwill, in order to do our best job. We can survive not being on the pedestal, however gloomily and reluctantly we may step down, but we can't survive being in the sewer.

Compassion in the examining room and clinic and hospital is impossible without mutual respect. Inevitably, this requires changes in physicians and the way we are trained, how we behave and the tasks we are expected to perform. But some changes are required of patients as well, if they are to receive the respect they so badly want in return.

All of us need to accept that there has been entirely too much concocted disease, that too much suffering and deviance has been defined as illness, and that not only physicians have profited from such convenient distortions. Virtually every day, I see a dozen or more patients who have come to see me primarily because they are unwilling to take responsibility for health problems that are easily within their competence, if only they had taken the time to read the most elementary first-aid books. They come to see me in part because they are lazy or fearful, and in part because of a vast regulatory system which makes "a visit to a physician" a required part of litigation, arbitration, and administrative processing.

I don't like being a part of such processes. I don't like what it does to me and to my patients and to the relationship we share. We need to abandon adversary postures, when such stances lead us to demean the efforts and character of persons with whom we have a shared task. We need to approach one another alert to virtues as well as to flaws. We have been obsessed by our demands for perfection and have been unforgiving of flaws and errors. We have failed to accept complexity, labeling deviations from perfection in patients as disease, and punishing deviations from perfection in otherwise competent physicians with malpractice suits and ridicule. We need to look at specific qualities of people, both positive and negative, but we need also to look beyond the specifics and weigh people in the aggregate.

We physicians have often been romantics, dedicated and selfless on the one hand, and subjective, idiosyncratic, and self-indulgent on the other. Like all romantics after the fantasies have withered in the glare of reality, we are left with disillusionment, a distress intensified by our sense of loneliness, and an uneasiness that no one understands or would be sympathetic. We see ourselves as tragic figures, like a priest who embraces his social function but who no longer believes in God—and who must keep his own counsel so that he may continue to serve parishioners who still cling to their faith. Feeling naked, often hypocritical, conscious of our own blunders and those of the institutions in which we serve, we struggle with our conscience and with our dedication. The burden of our doubts is sometimes overwhelming, but the price of certainty is a closed mind. Most of us nonetheless continue to do what we have been trained to do. What are the alternatives?

The romance is over, dead. That's part of what I think killed Alex and others. They came to medicine and psychiatry with a suitor's love. As the most ardent of romantics, they gave their all, but their love was unrequited. They sought an affair of the heart, and found instead a job, which was too often dreary, impersonal, numbing to the physician and injurious to the patient. Like Chris, they wanted to feel like knights errant, to be part of a greater order of aspiration; but unlike him, they ended up feeling like cogs, lacking impact, perceiving themselves as unloved and unworthy of love. They had such glowing expectations, so few of which materialized. They couldn't believe that the object of their love—the profession of medicine—was flawed in any significant way, so they blamed themselves and felt unworthy to continue.

Medicine goes on and psychiatry goes on, but the glow is gone. Some of my colleagues have died, and others will continue to die, because clinical work can become unendurable without a romantic's acceptance, optimism, and givingness.

Others have chosen different responses.

Some like Rose flee from patients altogether—into administration or research or processing paper for an insurance or pharmaceutical company or some governmental bureau. Others like Chris flee from the masses of sick and supposedly sick patients who demand so much and give so little, and practice instead in restrictive settings where they can nurture and protect a romantic style of patient care separate from more public pressures.

Some flee internally, performing little mental shifts which help make intolerable situations more livable. They make the compromises which are familiar to all of us in stereotype, and which help to fuel the public anger directed at the medical profession.

In recognizing the impossibility of always placing the patient's welfare primary, some do an about-face and consistently place their own interests before the patient's. Like disenchanted lovers, they become self-interested and calloused, always concerned about protecting themselves above all, focusing on their own security as their most important value. They are afraid to do otherwise. They take no risks on the patient's behalf, and dare not chance empathy, for it would make their own position untenable. They do their job at a minimal level as long as their own security demands it, or, if they can, perhaps do nothing at all, superficially content with a life of coffee breaks and absenteeism, seeking satisfaction in private rather than professional life. Sour-faced, bored, and unhappy, they do poor work and know it, but continue in their clinical roles because they can't believe that anything else would be better.

Others become angry and cynical and nihilistic. "Why do anything?" they ask. "None of it makes any difference anyhow." In stumbling on their own impotence in the face of the impossible demands of their profession, they become undermining of others who still have the energy to try. They decry romance in medicine when they see it; they have been too badly hurt to allow it in others. They dare not risk empathy with the patients either; for if they do, the patients' needs will overwhelm them. Instead, they create distance between themselves and the people seeking health care. Some doctors will use derogatory labels for their patients. Others will use pseudo-diagnostic labels—calling patients with emotional needs "dependency problems" or people who object to being processed "character disorders," finding protection in these abstractions, blaming the patients for the frustrations that have become inherent in the system.

Some seek succor in a rigid and authoritarian stance, because the stresses of medical practice are only tolerable as long as they can maintain some control. They cling to a mantle of cranky infallibility, because it is the only thing that keeps them from being overwhelmed by the cold wind of misery which buffets them daily in their professional practice. They adhere to the objective, the rational, the dispassionate. When they feel pain or entertain doubts, they stifle them. Their facade must be absolute, even to themselves. The recognition of fallibility and vulnerability is regarded as weakness, an intolerable assault on the self-perceived strength that fuels them in their clinical tasks.

And some—those for whom compromise or escape is simply not tolerable—work themselves to death, perhaps destroying others they love in the process, trying to be worthy of their romantic heritage.

They are all wounded healers, and so am I.

It helps me a bit to understand the problem and my own wounds more broadly than I did before I began this book. I feel less despondent and frustrated at my own inability to measure up to traditional expectations, and I am not quite so angry at patients when they ask me—either directly or by implication—for more than I feel I have to give.

Still, that anger is there, close to the surface; and still I feel guilty. I rationalize my limitations, but in my physician's soul, the romantic ideals live an enduring life. Deep inside, I continue to believe that physicians should embody all the wonderful qualities that romantics once attributed to them. Deep inside, when a patient's words or manner or behavior imply that I and my colleagues have wrongfully forsaken our heritage, I feel guilty. I feel powerless to change, but I feel guilty.

When students come to me for guidance in their own care of patients, I can only tell them that I am struggling too. I don't know any magic answers. The future looks pretty bleak for would-be healers. We simply have to do the best we can. The only advice I can give, I tell them, is to treat the patient with respect, and to try to maintain your self-respect as well. Try to marvel at the extraordinary range of behaviors human beings have for adapting to stress. Use your privileged contact with people to gain insights into human character and the human condition, but try not to get bogged down by all the pettiness and selfishness and conflicting bureaucratic pressures. Be alert to nobility in yourself and your patients and colleagues. Look for valor. If you don't look for it, you probably won't see it; and then you'll feel impossibly burdened by disease and suffering and your unbelievable responsibilities.

When I am lucky, I can see beyond all the complaints and problems—the earaches and tummyaches, the cuts and bruises, the runny noses and bladder infections, the twisted ankles and ingrown nails, the venereal disease and return-to-work slips—beyond all those things to the drama of people struggling to live their lives despite adversity. I try to ally myself with the forces of integration and healing, against the forces of disintegration and disease. I try to remain the patient's cheerful and creative ally, no matter how many pressures work to separate us. And I try to understand myself better in the process. Opportunities for nonexploitive self-revelation and self-discovery abound in medicine; and, if one is lucky, it's possible to find a nobler and wiser and more generous self.

Sometimes there are moments so sublime that I feel myself transcending all the pettiness and frustration. I never fail to be moved by the trust and privilege and magic inherent in that moment when I put my hand inside a woman in labor and feel the baby's head pushing down at me. Other times, when I use an ophthalmoscope and peek at the blood vessels pulsing in the hidden inner recesses of someone's eye, or read a cardiogram revealing the secret currents of a person's heart, or listen to the private turmoils that someone in agony will reveal only to a trusted physician—at these moments, I feel suddenly serene and wonderfully integrated with the excitement of the life that throbs around me. My wounds become my spectacles, helping me to see what I encounter with empathy and a grateful sense of privilege.

What is at issue for physicians is how we cope with wounding, and what we can learn from it, whether the process helps us to empathize with our patients and gives us an additional resource for healing them—or whether it drives us from them.

When we can, we must try to let our patients help us, by letting them know how hard we are struggling and with which forces. We must ask for their tolerance and compassion even as they seek these qualities from us. Our patients are often far stronger than our paternalistic heritage would lead us to believe, and they will often assist us once they understand our quandary.

Healing can be reciprocal, if we let it.

Notes

1. ALEX: The "Impaired Physician"

Since suicide by psychiatrists has become a growing problem, the professional literature is now starting to feature articles about how individual patients react to the suicide of their own therapists (see James C. Ballenger, "Patients' Reactions to the Suicide of Their Psychiatrist," *Journal of Nervous and Mental Disease,* vol. 166, pp. 859–67, December 1978). The problem is not a new one, however; a number of Freud's close early colleagues killed themselves, including Paul Federn, Wilhelm Stekel, and Viktor Tausk (Part 7, "Mortido—The Death Instinct," in Walter Freeman, *The Psychiatrist—Personalities and Patterns,* New York, Grune and Stratton, 1968). Some people think that depression is a predictable human response for most people who become psychiatrists (Berl Mendel, "On Therapist Watching," *Psychiatry,* vol. 27, pp. 59–68, February 1964). No matter how predictable, however, suicides by gifted people, capable of substantial contributions to their community, are deeply troubling, especially when they occur among those who are young and still in training (Robert Pasnau and Andrew Russell, "Psychiatric Resident Suicide—An Analysis of Five Cases," *American Journal of Psychiatry,* pp. 402–406, April 1975).

The literature on nonpsychiatric physicians in trouble is voluminous but generally suffers from a tendency to describe the phenomenon in disease terms. Michael a'Brook and colleagues wrote what is still one of the better articles of this genre (M. F. a'Brook et al., "Psychiatric Illness in the Medical Profession," *British Journal of Psychiatry,* vol. 113, pp. 1013–23, 1967). Ross's paper is likewise worth reading (Mathew Ross, "Suicide Among Physicians," *Psychiatry in*

Medicine, vol. 2, pp. 189–198, July 1971). As an index of how widespread is the problem of doctors coping successfully with stress, one article maintains that "the chances of becoming a drug addict are higher for doctors than for ghetto youths" (Michael Rosenbaum, "The Screaming Silence of the Disabled Physician," *Medical Dimensions,* pp. 23–31, February 1976). Anyone interested in keeping abreast of current information concerning the impaired physician issue would do well to read the "American Medical Association Impaired Physician Newsletter," available from the American Medical Association in Chicago. The same organization also produces lengthy monographs detailing the proceedings of their Annual Conferences on the Impaired Physician. Published papers that view the same phenomenon from other than a disease perspective remain the exception (Howard Grindlinger, "Out of Touch—Medicine as an Impaired Profession," *Medical Dimensions,* pp. 36–37, December 1978/January 1979).

5. THE DOCTOR-PATIENT RELATIONSHIP: Setting Emotional Limits

Articles that discuss the impact of a patient's death, especially suicide, on the patient's physician are relatively less numerous than one would suppose. Litman's paper reports the results of interviews with two hundred psychotherapists (R. E. Litman, "When Patients Commit Suicide," *Journal of Psychotherapy,* vol. 19, pp. 570–76, 1965). A more recent paper has dealt with the phenomenon as experienced by therapists in training (Susan Kolodney et al., "The Working Through of Patients' Suicides by Four Therapists," *Suicide and Life-Threatening Behavior,* vol. 9, pp. 33–46, Spring 1979).

Chapman provides an interesting personal perspective, which reflects the luxury of choices available to a popular private practitioner: "I haven't had any suicides in the past three years and only one in the past five years. It's not because I've grown wiser, but because I avoid risky cases, like the wrist slasher I sent to [another younger psychiatrist] today. As I grow older and my own death draws nearer, I become too painfully anxious when a patient destroys himself because I didn't pick up the right clues, or was careless, or erred in my judgment, or, perhaps, had bad luck." (A. H. Chapman, *It's All Arranged—Fifteen Hours in a Psychiatrist's Life,* New York, Putnam, 1975.)

For the nonpsychiatric medical practitioners, death generally becomes a more constant companion as the physician's age increases. When patients have the opportunity to choose, young physicians tend to attract young patients. As the doctor ages, his patients age with him; so that older practitioners tend to have many dying patients whom they have known and cared for over many years. Several older internist friends carry this burden lovingly, but it is a burden nonetheless.

7. THE DOCTOR-PATIENT RELATIONSHIP: In Pursuit of Integration

That Sallie's experience with addicts is not unique has been well documented (Leon Wurmser, "Drug Abuse—Nemesis of Psychiatry," *The American Scholar,* vol. 41, pp. 393–407, Summer 1972). Many would say that such frustrating and ultimately misguided attempts at healing are a natural consequence of "grandiose claims of psychiatry's ability to right social wrongs, . . . [and] the perceived lack of scientific underpinnings of the discipline . . ." (Peter Bourne, "The Psychiatrist's Responsibility and the Public Trust," *American Journal of Psychiatry,* vol. 135, pp. 174–177, February 1978). In attempting to right social wrongs, psychiatry has often wandered far from areas of clearly defined competence (see, for example, S. H. Kaufman, "Prejudice as a Sociopsychiatric Responsibility," *American Journal of Psychiatry,* vol. 104, pp. 44–47, 1947, and Roy Grinker, "Psychiatry Rides Madly in All Directions," *Archives of General Psychiatry,* vol. 10, pp. 228–37, 1964). Dumont provides one highly personal account of the community psychiatry movement, which transformed many psychiatrists from healers of the soul to awkward and often impotent healers of society (Matthew Dumont, *The Absurd Healer—Perspectives of a Community Psychiatrist,* New York, Science House, 1968).

The same thing of course has happened with medicine generally: "Medicine has always displayed an eagerness to appropriate many of mankind's vast panoply of problems, especially if they can be transliterated into medical nomenclature. When therapeutic success eluded such practitioners, they simply redoubled their efforts. This phenomenon has been labeled 'creeping medical imperialism' " (Lloyd Sederer, "Moral Therapy and the Problem of Morale," *American Journal of Psychiatry,* vol. 134, pp. 267–272, March 1979).

The growth of cynicism in medical students has been the subject of considerable attention in the literature. Eron contributed an early report (Leonard Eron, "Effect of Medical Education on Medical Students' Attitudes," *Journal of Medical Education,* vol. 30, pp. 559–566, October 1955). Becker and Geer noted the same phenomenon, but called it realism (H. F. Becker and B. Geer, "The Fate of Idealism in Medical School," *American Sociological Review,* vol. 28, pp. 70–80, 1958), whereas Coker and associates say "Machiavellianism" (R. E. Coker, et al., "Authoritarianism and Machiavellianism Among Medical Students," *Journal of Medical Education,* vol. 40, pp. 1074–84, 1965). Keniston, in a classic article on medical students, maintains that "to attempt to retain human sensitivity . . . in the modern world is to oppose many of the most powerful trends in our society; it is obviously not easy" (Kenneth Keniston, "The Medical Student," *World Journal of Biology and Medicine,* vol. 39, pp. 346–58, 1967). Halberstam talks about his clinical teaching, wherein he bombards students with his own boundless enthusiasm, and concludes that "our fine young recruits are coming into the profession, not with a feeling of exhilaration, but with a sense of foreboding" (Michael J. Halberstam, "Fear and Loathing in the Freshman Class," *Modern Medicine,* pp. 13–18, December 15, 1978).

Tension between science and art in medicine has been the subject of hundreds, perhaps thousands, of mostly thoughtful discourses. Sanazaro provides a good introduction to the literature (Paul J. Sanazaro, "Innovations in Medical Education—Social and Scientific Determinants," *Archives of Neurology,* vol. 17, pp. 484–493, November 1967). Blackwell maintains that the tension can easily result in polarization of medical-school faculties, with so-called humanists feeling "academically overwhelmed" and scientists becoming "emotionally exacerbated" (Barry Blackwell et al., "Humanizing the Student-Cadaver Encounter," presented at the annual meeting of the American Psychiatric Association, May 16, 1979). Knight, in what is a generally sanguine tribute to medical students and medicine, occasionally lapses into gloomy fatalism, saying for instance that "students are often told on the day of entering medical school that when the sun goes down, they will be far behind in their work and will never catch up in their lifetime" (James A. Knight, *Medical Student—Doctor in the Making,* New York, Appleton-Century-Croft, 1973).

May analyzes his own experience as a medical student and discusses the problem in terms of gender, citing a predominance of "male principles" over "female principles" (Scott May, "On My Medical Education—Seeking a Balance in Medicine," *Medical Self-Care,* No. 5, pp. 37–41, 1979). Werner and Korsch try to maintain optimism and remain cautionary at the same time, stressing that "the development of the empathic relationship is one of the most difficult processes in medical professionalization" (Edwenna Werner and Barbara Korsch, "The Vulnerability of the Medical Student—Posthumous Presentation of L. L. Stephens' Ideas," *Pediatrics,* vol. 57, pp. 321–28, 1976). Pilowsky takes a balanced, anthropologic approach and concludes that "the community need to perceive doctors as altruistic, alternates with the need to condemn them as self-seeking, just as doctors vary in their perceptions of patients from being worthy recipients of aid to being undeserving 'cheaters.' This conflict between man and his appointed helpers is as old as man himself, and must, it would seem, be regarded as an inevitable consequence of his very nature" (Issy Pilowsky, "Altruism and the Practice of Medicine," *British Journal of Medical Psychology,* vol. 50, pp. 305–11, 1977).

While psychiatry's denotative role has been caring for mental illness, its connotative role, especially in the medical schools, has been the nurturance of compassion and other human sensibilities among medical professionals. Some assertions by the profession's leaders have been positively messianic. White, for example, effused "that psychiatry is the one medical specialty which in its broadest conception can be seen to be the central point of all the other medical specialties; for it is only from the standpoint of the psychiatrist, or perhaps better, from the psychological level, that the significance of disease of the various parts of the body can be understood" (William White, *Twentieth-Century Psychiatry,* New York, W. W. Norton and Company, 1936). Ebaugh and Rymer, writing in a book that was to be influential in medical-school curriculum design, exclaimed that "the medical course ought to convey more competence in dealing with the total personality and that this can be realized through more training in psychiatry" (Franklin Ebaugh and Charles Rymer, *Psychiatry in Medical Education,* New York, The Commonwealth Fund, 1942). Whitehorn and associates echoed the same message, solidifying a role which psychiatry has maintained to the present day: "The aim of psychiatric teaching in the medical school is to prepare the medical student to deal intelligently and skillfully with patients as persons, and to provide him with the basic knowledge of psychological and social problems and resources in relation to health and disease" (John Whitehorn, et al., *Psychiatry in Medical Education,* Washington, D.C., American Psychiatric Association, 1952; see also John Romano, "The Teaching of Psychiatry to Medical Students Past, Present, and Future," *American Journal of Psychiatry,* vol. 26, pp. 1115–1126, February 1970).

Useful overviews of the consultation-liaison approach include Pasnau (Robert Pasnau, *Consultation-Liaison Psychiatry,* New York, Grune and Stratton, 1975) and more recently Faguet (Roert Faguet, et al., *Contemporary Models in Liaison Psychiatry,* New York, SP Medical and Scientific Books, 1978). A somewhat more jaundiced view by a battered and bruised veteran of consultation-liaison teaching can be seen in a seldom-quoted article by McKegney (F. Patrick McKegney, "Consultation-Liaison Teaching of Psychosomatic Medicine—Opportunities and Obstacles," *Journal of Nervous and Mental Disease,* vol. 154, pp. 198–205, 1972).

8. IRV: Out of Step

For me, the literature on quality control in medicine is difficult to read and depressing. Most of the primary sources, including the governmental statutes and administrative guidelines remain on my shelf unread, despite numerous good-faith attempts. The American Psychiatric Association has a tolerable pamphlet on the subject as it relates to psychiatry (Robert Gibson, ed., *Professional Responsibilities and Peer Review in Psychiatry,* Washington, D.C., American Psychiatric Association, 1977). Towery and Sharfstein focus on one of the economic rationales for "quality-control efforts" (O. B. Towery and Steven Sharfstein, "Fraud and Abuse in Psychiatric Practice," *American Journal of Psychiatry,* vol. 135, pp. 92–94, January 1978), while Towery and Windle review the pivotal 1975 amendments (O. B. Towery and Charles Windle, "Quality Assurance for Community Mental Health Centers—Impact of P.L. 94–63," *Hospital and Community Psychiatry,* vol. 29, pp. 316–319, May 1978). Sullivan observes that physicians are "always slow to grasp external reality" and concludes with the widely touted prediction that "lack of involvement [by physicians] will only ensure continued design of review procedures by eager and willing others" (Frank Sullivan, "Peer Review and PSRO—An Update," *American Journal of Psychiatry,* vol. 133, pp. 51–54, January 1976). Shwed and co-workers provide one of many cautionary articles about the impact of quality-care audits on essential trust between doctor and patient (Shwed, et al., "Medicaid Audit—Crisis in Confidentiality and the Patient-Psychiatrist Relationship," *American Journal of Psychiatry,* vol. 136, pp. 447–450, April 1979). My own enthusiastic but embarrassingly naïve contribution to the quality-care literature has long since been outdated (Martin Lipp, "Quality Control in Psychiatry and the Problem-Oriented System," *International Journal of Psychiatry,* vol. 11, pp. 355–381, 1973).

9. THE DOCTOR-PATIENT RELATIONSHIP: Documenting Competence

A previous article of mine addresses the issue of motivation in caring for the chronically ill (Martin Lipp, "What's in It for the Therapist?" *Hospital and Community Psychiatry,* vol. 29, pp. 40–41, January 1978).

The declining number of physicians going into office-based, as opposed to institutionally based, practice may be followed in publications produced at regular intervals by the American Medical Association (see, e.g., Sharon Henderson, ed., *Profile of Medical Practice,* 1977 edition, Chicago, Ill., American Medical Association, 1977). Stalker notes that "the number of available office-based primary-care practitioners has taken a whopping nosedive—from 110,000 down to 53,000—over a 20-year period from 1950 to 1972." He concludes by saying that "for millions of Americans, hospitals have become sources of primary care assistance by choice. What Sears and Roebuck Company was to rural America in the 1920s, '30s, and '40s, hospitals, especially community hospitals in metropolitan areas—where the majority of residents train—have evolved into centers of medical care which offer all things to all people (Timothy Stalker, "What's Behind the Explosive Growth in Hospital-Based Primary Care?" *Hospital Physician,* vol. 15, pp. 26–29, February 1979).

Funkenstein has reported on trends away from solo practice among graduates from Harvard Medical School over an eighteen-year period, from 1958 to 1976: "The significant change in lifestyle is that [now] nearly all students wish to work fewer hours and to have more time for their families and outside activities. This they see as best accomplished by group practice, and over 95 percent of the students currently plan this type of practice." He adds parenthetically that "only secondarily do they see group practice as a means for improving the quality or lowering the cost of medical care" (Daniel Funkenstein, Sr., *Medical Students, Medical Schools and Society During Five Eras*, Cambridge, Mass., Ballinger Publishing, 1978).

The expanding role of science, as opposed to art, in psychiatry is a fascinating topic in itself, too complex to go into here. However, one landmark may be of interest. On July 1, 1947, the National Institute of Mental Health made available funds for its first research grant, MH-1-RO1, based on a proposal to study "the basic nature of the learning process—neurological aspects." The bland title, suggesting observations derived from classrooms or clinics, may be deceptive. The experiment actually involved conditioning nine dogs with electrical shocks, operating on six to remove half their brains, and finally subjecting all nine dogs to further testing. Maybe it was an omen. Readers interested in personally assessing the results of grant MH-1 will find information a matter of public record (W. N. Kellogg, "Locomotor and Other Disturbances Following Hemidecortication in the Dog," *The Journal of Comparative and Physiological Psychology*, vol. 6, pp. 506–516, December 1949).

Auden's line about scientists is from a volume of his collected essays (W. H. Auden, *The Dyer's Hand and Other Essays*, New York, Random House, 1948).

More information on the experience of being a board exam casualty is available in the professional literature (see, e.g., Martin Lipp, "Experiences of Psychiatry Board Exam Casualties—A Survey Report," *American Journal of Psychiatry*, vol. 133, pp. 279–283, March 1976).

10. RUSSELL: The Shock Doctor

The Snake Pit, many readers will know, is a classic and fascinating first-person account of insanity and hospitalization (Mary Jane Ward, *The Snake Pit*, New York, Random House, 1946).

"The Shock Doctor Register" is a regular feature of *Madness Network News*, "a quarterly journal of psychiatric inmates/antipsychiatry movement" (see, e.g., vol. 5, no. 4, p. 18, Spring 1979).

The special psychological needs and stresses of the physician's family have been the subject of a growing literature. The Crays, husband and wife, deal specifically with the issue of "patient envy" (Cameron Cray and Marjorie Cray, "Stresses and Rewards Within the Psychiatrist's Family," *American Journal of Psychoanalysis,* vol. 37, pp. 337–41, 1977). One article by a physician's wife, subtitled "Isn't Marriage to God on Earth Enough?" examines evolving trends (Barbara Seaman, "The Changing Lives of (Some) Doctors' Wives," *Medical Dimensions,* pp. 19–30, February 1975). Growing resentment by spouses of physicians' devotion to work and patients is an increasingly common topic in the medical press (see, e.g., "Doctors' Wives Give Vent to Their Feelings of Neglect," *Medical Tribune,* August 23, 1978).

The impact of rules and regulations on physician behavior has not been fully comprehended, and I have not been able to find any comprehensive treatments of the subject. However, numerous articles deal with fragments of the problem. Fleischman pleads for the right to retain discretion in clinical practice, saying "if we punish fallibility—as we do when the malpractice lawyer becomes our regulatory agency—then we have destroyed medicine. The climate in which we practice must allow us to attempt innovations, and even fail at 'routines,' since ultimately the best medical practice rests on the perception that nothing is routine and that each event is a unique combination of circumstances. To be able to stand uncertain and searching in the midst of our patients' dilemmas is the essence of psychiatry" (Paul Fleischman, "Regulating Psychiatric Practice," *American Journal of Psychiatry,* vol. 134, pp. 296–298, March 1977). Trainer has quoted physician-attorney Walter Feldman as saying "good medicine cannot survive the erosion of professional discretion now taking place. Its replacement by judicial fiat is not the answer. Clinical variables require choices based on skill and discretion, not legal pronouncements" (Dorothy Trainer, "Psychiatrists Said Mistrusted—Professional Discretion Eroding," *Psychiatric News,* p. 3, December 1, 1978).

Alan Stone, president of the American Psychiatric Association from 1979 to 1980, has contributed some of the more readable and thoughtful commentary concerning these trends, including the Donaldson decision (see, e.g., Alan Stone, "Overview: The Right to Treatment, Comments on the Law and Its Impact," *American Journal of Psychiatry,* vol. 132, pp. 1125–34, November 1975, and "Recent Mental Health Litigation—A Critical Perspective," *American Journal of Psychiatry,* vol. 134, pp. 273–280, March 1977). *O'Connor* v. *Donald-*

son refers to a U.S. Supreme Court ruling in June 1975 which holds that a patient who is not dangerous to self or others must be discharged from custodial care if he is not being actively treated and if he can survive "safely" in freedom. Thus, a chronically ill, marginally or intermittently self-sufficient individual—who could be expected to gravitate to a skid-row existence or whose home care would create an intolerable burden on a family—cannot be involuntarily confined in an institution if treatment makes no difference in his basic condition. The journal *Drug Therapy* has produced a special issue, providing a useful overview which gives some idea of the range of issues involved in the more narrow topic of drug prescribing alone (Ray Gifford, Jr., guest ed., "Regulating the Practice of Medicine," *Drug Therapy,* December 1978).

The issue of involuntary medicating has come up in many states other than Massachusetts. A class-action suit initiated in California named Governor Jerry Brown and other state officials as defendants in what was termed "chemical rape" ("Mental Patients Sue to Refuse Dangerous Drugs," *ACLU News,* vol. 43, pp. 1–3, March 1978).

Angry arguments about shock therapy have also consumed a good deal of newsprint. A reasonably balanced account can be found in *Psychiatric News* (see Margaret McDonald's two-part series, "The ECT Controversy," *Psychiatric News,* January and February 1977).

11. THE DOCTOR-PATIENT RELATIONSHIP: Assembly-Line Medicine

Medicine is not the only profession to become an assembly-line phenomenon. California Supreme Court Justice Rose Bird has said that "the American judicial system now resembles an assembly line in which people become inanimate objects to be processed." She noted that not only the public is demeaned in the process: "Judges too become grist for the computer mill, as they are transformed into 'judicial position equivalents' and their work into 'average minutes involved per filing' for the purpose of cranking out 'weighted work load' results" (William Moore, "Bird Calls It Assembly-Line Justice," San Francisco *Chronicle,* p. 10, January 24, 1978).

Levitt has written a fascinating and revealing paper arguing for the application of assembly-line principles to service industries. Citing McDonald's hamburgers as an example, he maintains that "discretion is the enemy of order, standardization and quality" (Theodore

Levitt, "Production-Line Approach to Service," *Harvard Business Review,* vol. 50, pp. 41–52, September–October 1972).

For a newsy overview on the topic of measuring productivity of health-care workers, including physicians, see the account by Rhein (Reginald Rhein, Jr., "Measuring Physicians' Productivity," *Medical World News,* pp. 37–44, April 16, 1979).

The rent-a-doc phenomenon is spreading. The Western Physicians Medical Group, which services Alturas, California, also supplies rotating physicians to three other communities in northern California and Nevada (Dianne Hales, "Rx for Rural Areas: Rent-A-Doc," *Impact/American Medical News,* pp. 6–7, December 22, 1978). Emergency Med-Phone connects patients by phone with doctors they have never seen for instant advice. The service, which charges individuals $25 per year plus $2.50 per call, was designed to meet a perceived need: over half the people in New York City do not have their own physician (Wendy Grabel, "Dial-A-Doc Service Debuts to Criticism in New York," *Medical Tribune,* p. 17, July 4, 1979).

12. WARREN: Doctor or Double Agent

Mawardi's longitudinal career studies of physician graduates from Case Western Reserve revealed that not only Warren is frightened by his patients: "One could scarcely believe it when it was learned that physicians feared violence against themselves and their families from disgruntled patients.... This fear has become a new or more prevalent stress in physicians" (Betty Mawardi, "Satisfactions, Dissatisfactions, and Causes of Stress in Medical Practice," *JAMA,* pp. 1483–1486, April 6, 1979).

With regard to child abuse, Savage reports that "the physician who fails to file . . . a report would be exposed to civil liability for professional malpractice when failure to report leads to continued child abuse. At least 37 states provide for criminal penalties for physicians who fail to report battered children" (Douglas Savage, "The Physician's Duty to Report Battered Child Syndrome," *The Journal of Family Practice,* vol. 9, pp. 429–40, 1979).

Newberger and Bourne provide a review of child-abuse literature; but, like many of us, they are more helpful in analyzing the present state of affairs than in saying how it should be different (Eli Newberger and Richard Bourne, "The Medicalization and Legalization of

Child Abuse," *American Journal of Orthopsychiatry,* vol. 48, pp. 593–607, October 1978). Conrad, in a related article, does an excellent sociological assessment of hyperkinesis as a medical phenomenon, speculating that perhaps the availability of new social control mechanisms leads to new medical labels (Peter Conrad, "The Discovery of Hyperkinesis: Notes on the Medicalization of Deviant Behavior," *Social Problems,* vol. 23, p. 12–21, 1975).

Ben-David wrote one of the earliest articles on physicians torn between obligations to employer and patient (J. Ben-David, "The Professional Role of the Physician in Bureaucratized Medicine—A Study in Role Conflict," *Human Relations,* vol. 11, pp. 255–74, 1958). Daniels investigated the dilemmas faced by the psychiatrist in such a situation, and published her findings with a scholarly sociological analysis (A. K. Daniels, "The Captive Professional—Bureaucratic Limitations in the Practice of Military Psychiatry," *Journal of Health and Social Behavior,* vol. 10, pp. 255–65, 1969). A decade later, the published transcript of a Conference on Conflicting Loyalties added still more perspective ("In the Service of the State: The Psychiatrist as Double Agent," a report of the Conference on Conflicting Loyalties, co-sponsored by the American Psychiatric Association and the Hastings Center, March 24–26, 1977). The topic has also received attention in the psychoanalytic literature (Arnold Gilberg, "A Psychoanalyst: An Agent of the Social Milieu," *American Journal of Psychoanalysis,* vol. 36, pp. 325–29, 1976) and the popular press (Fred Powledge, "The Therapist as Double Agent," *Psychology Today,* pp. 44–47, July 1977).

The adversary relationship between doctors and patients, such as it is, increasingly is being shepherded by attorneys. Weitzel has reviewed some of the relevant literature and concluded that "psychiatrists are ill equipped to reliably interpret evolving mental health law. Psychiatric facilities should retain skilled counsel on call to consult with psychiatrists at the time questions arise. Hours of unproductive worry and well-meaning but potentially expensive legal blunders by psychiatrists could thus be avoided" (William Weitzel, "Changing Law and Clinical Dilemmas," *American Journal of Psychiatry,* vol. 134, March 1977).

Alan Stone provides a similar perspective: "The idea of having a legal advocate representing every mental patient is all right . . . but only if the psychiatrist also has a legal representative" ("Stone Says

Psychiatry Needs Own Advocate," *Psychiatric News,* p. 3, October 19, 1979).

For an angry civil-liberty lawyer's view of these issues, see Ennis's autobiographical account (Bruce Ennis, *Prisoners of Psychiatry,* New York, Harcourt Brace Jovanovich, 1972). Rothman provides a more balanced perspective, pointing out that "there now exists a widespread and acute suspicion of the very notion of doing good among widely divergent groups on all points of the political spectrum. To claim to act for the purposes of benevolence was once sufficient to legitimate a program; at this moment it is certain to create suspicion. ... The commitment to paternalistic state intervention in the name of equality is giving way to a commitment to restrict intervention in the name of liberty" (David Rothman in Willard Gaylin, et al., *Doing Good—The Limits of Benevolence,* New York, Pantheon, 1978).

Simultaneously with the increasing interest in physicians' conflicting roles, there has been a growing number of articles that reflect the diversity of emotions experienced by such physicians, as well as a spreading disenchantment with some patients (see, e.g., James Groves, "Taking Care of the Hateful Patient," *New England Journal of Medicine,* vol. 298, pp. 883–87, 1978; Jean Goodwin, et al., "Psychiatric Symptoms in Disliked Medical Patients," *Journal of the American Medical Association,* vol. 241, pp. 1117–1120, March 16, 1979; John Maltsberger and Dan Buie, "Countertransference Hate in the Treatment of Suicidal Patients," *Archives of General Psychiatry,* vol. 30, pp. 625–633, May 1974; Victor Altschul, "The So-Called Boring Patient," *American Journal of Psychotherapy,* pp. 533–545, vol. 31, October 1977; Bess Udell and Robijn Hornstra, "Good Patients and Bad—Therapeutic Assets and Liabilities," *Archives of General Psychiatry,* vol. 32, pp. 1533–1537, December 1975).

Onion, an internist and associate medical director of a rural health program, observes: "Most of us who enter medicine, and especially those in primary care specialties, do so with idealistic goals of serving humankind. ... At the same time, most of us hope to preserve our own humanity. Most of us fail. ... It is a rare doc, at least among those on the primary care front lines, who is not burdened with substantial anger, and guilt about the anger" (Daniel K. Onion, "Physicians' Lib," *Forum on Medicine,* p. 266, April 1979). Norman, in another context, is philosophical about such feelings in a surgeon friend:

"I figured that bartenders and doctors see the worst in people and that either you catch the hating disease or you don't" (Geoffrey Norman, "Comfort Me with Leaves," *Esquire,* pp. 92–93, October 1979).

My own book, I think, puts the issue of why doctors and patients are sometimes at odds in a balanced perspective (see Ch. 8, "Problem Patients," Martin Lipp, *Respectful Treatment: The Human Side of Medical Care,* Hagerstown, Md., Harper & Row, 1977).

13. THE DOCTOR-PATIENT RELATIONSHIP: Conflicting Allegiances

With regard to reportable diseases, the onus is increasingly on the physician. For example, in the instance of a patient having a single lapse of consciousness, "unless the physician can categorically state that the condition cannot possibly cause recurrent lapses, it should be reported" (*Action Report,* Board of Medical Quality Assurance, State of California, April 1979).

There is a growing skepticism that some "public health" requirements serve primarily to increase bureaucratic funding or at least to preserve bureaucratic organizations. On a related issue, Imperato points out that "every year for the past several years, zealous public health officials have forecast serious epidemics of measles, polio, diphtheria, and pertussis.... The epidemics and other dire consequences that have been predicted for the past several years have not materialized in the public's view ... and the incident has served only to reinforce the public's skepticism of statements made by public health officials about other communicable diseases" (P. J. Imperato, "Immunization in an Era of Skepticism," *Drug Therapy,* vol. 7, pp. 22–23, October 1977).

That doctors have responsibilities to the employers of their patients is not simply a quirk of chance. "Employers picked up the tab for about 40 billion dollars of the nation's 183 billion dollars in health care expenses in 1978. In fact, employee medical benefit costs have risen so rapidly that they account for as much as 10 percent of total compensation in some companies. This alarming trend has persuaded many large corporations to band together in regional groups to map cost-cutting strategies that may have greater impact than their individual efforts have achieved so far.... We have not begun to maximize the leverage warranted by the hundreds of millions of dollars we contribute annually to the health care providers. . . ." ("The Corporate Attack on Rising Medical Costs," *Business Week*, pp. 54–56, August 6, 1979).

The Tarasoff decision refers to a bizarre series of circumstances in which Tatiana Tarasoff was murdered by Prosenjiit Poddar, an exsuitor who had been a psychiatric outpatient at the University of California Health Clinic in Berkeley. Poddar's murderous impulses had come up in therapy and his therapist had notified the police, but not the intended victim herself. The patient dropped out of psychotherapy when the therapist tried to hospitalize him. The court described the therapist's actions as being "in careless disregard of the victim's life and safety." The resultant ruling "created a situation in which acceptance of a patient into therapy imposes on therapists the duty to care for both the patient and any potential victims of the patient's dangerous actions. Thus the therapist must warn authorities specified by the law as well as potential victims of possible dangerous actions of their patients" (Howard Gurevitz, "Tarasoff: Protective Privilege Versus Public Peril," *American Journal of Psychiatry*, vol. 134, pp. 289–292, March 1977). The entire episode has been the subject of a number of fascinating accounts (see, e.g., Margaret McDonald's three part retrospective analysis in the December 1976 and January 1977 issues of *Psychiatric News).*

Szasz's contributions are well known (see Thomas Szasz, *The Myth of Mental Illness,* New York, Harper & Row, 1961). The selection quoted in this chapter is taken from his introduction to Ennis's book (Bruce Ennis, *Prisoners of Psychiatry,* New York, Harcourt Brace Jovanovich, 1972).

The trend for physicians with administrative authority to leave patient care is well documented: "Two decades ago [physicians] were trained by a few charismatic, humanistic clinicians who did not have much to do with laboratories or fund raising. After World War II academic [medicine] was transformed, largely by federal money, into a multidimensional scientific enterprise, the leaders of which needed to be scientific entrepreneurs as well as persuasive humanists. But . . . since the fantastic promise of a technology for universal well-being could not be fulfilled before the sources of financial support began to dry up, departmental chairmen are evolving from humanistic scientists into corporate executives who haven't the time or energy to pursue clinical elegance . . . first hand" (Arnold Mandell, "The Changing

Face of Chairmen of Psychiatry Departments in America: An Opinion," *American Journal of Psychiatry*, vol. 131, pp. 1137–1139, October 1974).

14. ROSE: The Doctor with No Patients

For a highly readable account of the development of CMHCs, such as those where Warren and Rose work, see Bassuk and Gerson (Ellen Bassuk and Samuel Gerson, "Deinstitutionalization and Mental Health Services," *Scientific American*, vol. 238, pp. 46–53, February 1978). However, psychiatrists like Rose have been fleeing such institutions for a number of years (see Walter Winslow, "CMHCs: Where Have All the Psychiatrists Gone?" presented at the annual meeting of the American Psychiatric Association, Toronto, Canada, May 1977; and Paul Fink and Steven Weinstein, "Whatever Happened to Psychiatry? The Deprofessionalization of Community Mental Health Centers," *American Journal of Psychiatry*, vol. 136, pp. 406–409, April 1979). The same phenomenon has affected the state hospitals (Gabriel Koz, "The Exodus of Psychiatrists, Influx of Nonpsychiatrists," *Psychiatric Opinion*, vol. 15, pp. 33–35, October 1978). Greenbaum contributed an earlier and perceptive view of the "abandon ship" phenomenon (Marvin Greenbaum, "Resignations Among Professional Mental Health Leaders—A Study of a Mild Epidemic," *Archives of General Psychiatry*, vol. 19, pp. 266–28, September 1968). Cherniss and Egnatios studied 164 subjects in 22 different programs in Michigan, including psychiatrists, nurses, social workers, psychologists, and others, and found low satisfaction with the work itself (Cary Cherniss and Edward Egnatios, "Is There Job Satisfaction in Community Mental Health?" *Community Mental Health Journal*, vol. 14, pp. 309–18, 1978). Crippen, a surgeon, looks at nonpsychiatric physicians struggling in bureaucratized medicine, and worries that "any desire to treat the sick can't help but be replaced by contempt for the system and everyone in it—including the patient." He concludes that "doctors might begin to leave direct patient care altogether" (David Crippen, "Doctoring on Demand—Right Versus Privilege in Medicine," *Medical Dimensions*, pp. 32–37, April 1978). Support for his prognostication comes from various studies which have compared the amount of time doctors spend with patients in private practice as opposed to institutionalized practice. For instance, while the average private psychiatrist spends 88 percent of the work week seeing patients, psychiatrists in institutional settings spend only half their time seeing patients, and those in the most prestigious locations—the medical schools—spend only 20 percent of the average work week with patients (Franklyn Arnhoff and A. H. Kumbar, *The Nation's Psychiatrist—1970 Survey,* Washington, D.C., American Psychiatric Association, 1973). Kubie believes that the phenomenon is traceable to the medical schools themselves. He says "in all fields of medicine nonclinicians are being appointed to lead clinical departments. What is worse, young investigators from the basic sciences who are devoid of clinical experience of any kind are being appointed to posts where clinical experience is essential both for basic progress and for its human application. . . . These tendencies are further complicated by the fact that among the late-age dropouts from clinical work many turn bitterly against their earlier activities, misleading younger men into following suit. . . . These dropouts are symptoms of a new disease . . . a disease without a name whose presenting symptom is a retreat from patients not unlike the retreat of college faculties from their students" (Lawrence Kubie, "The Retreat from Patients—An Unanticipated Penalty of the Full-Time System," *Archives of General Psychiatry,* vol. 24, pp. 98–106, February 1971). He could have added that it is these dropouts who are most likely to go on to health-care policy-making positions, resulting in decisions that will drive still more clinicians from patient care.

The phenomenon is not limited to medicine; many occupations are similarly affected. One defense analyst plaintively describes the situation in the military: "Almost nobody is trained for combat any more. They're businessmen. Until we change that, nothing else will count" (Pierre Sprey, quoted in *The Atlantic,* October 1979, p. 63).

15. THE END OF "THE DOCTOR KNOWS BEST"

The extravagance of hopes attached to medicine in the early years of this century was so monumental that it is embarrassing to read today. Haggard wrote that "the physician of today, aided by science and industry, stands . . . upon the prow of the ship of civilization. No longer is he scanning the horizon for the site of sea monsters and other fabrications of mystery and magic. With chart in hand and scientific instruments of precision at his disposal he is piloting us toward the peaceful harbor of old age, undisturbed by the terrors which formerly haunted the most intrepid voyager on the sea of life" (Howard Haggard, *Mystery, Magic, and Medicine,* p. 149, New York, Doubleday Doran, 1933). Writing in the same year, Clendenning surveyed the future of medical practice and forecast with sublime optimism that "the only safe prediction is that there is no limit to the accomplishments possible" (Logan Clendenning, *The Romance of Medicine,* p. 445, New York, Garden City Publishing Co., 1933). Psychiatry's future seemed as bright as that of the rest of medicine, and some thought more so: "Psychiatry . . . probably enjoys a wider popular interest at the present time than does any other field of medicine" (William Menninger, *Psychiatry: Its Evolution and Present Status,* p. 2, Ithaca, N.Y., Cornell University Press, 1948). Even as late as 1960, Freeman and Small could write: "We can expect less delinquency and crime as psychoanalysis, which has just started to penetrate prison walls, is used more intensively to help men understand why they rebel. . . . Psychoanalytic treatment will also be used for drug addicts. . . . We can expect the law . . . to become less punitive. . . . We can expect newspapers to interpret what happens in the world with more understanding of the deeper motives of men. . . . We can expect, also, far less physical illness" (Lucy Freeman and Marvin Small, *The Story of Psychoanalysis,* pp. 162–163, New York, Pocket Books, 1960). Freeman, with a different co-author, was later to write the story of the first woman to successfully sue her psychiatrist for using sex in the guise of therapy (see Lucy Freeman and Julie Roy, *Betrayal,* New York, Stein and Day, 1976). Not only the patient had felt betrayed; Lucy Freeman had earlier co-authored yet another book with the same psychiatrist who was the subject of the suit.

The medicalization of human events and the concomitant popularization and vulgarization of medicine and psychiatry escalated dramatically in the postwar years (see chapter "The Psychology-Psychiatry Boom," in Ernest Havemann, *The Age of Psychology,* New York, Simon and Schuster, 1957).

In the mid-1960s there were seven regularly scheduled nationally televised dramas devoted to the role of medicine, hospitals, and doctors. Their popularity and ubiquitousness made medicine's most brilliant accomplishments and most arcane language seem familiar, even vapid. The physician became a prosaic creature, whose ability to cure primarily on the basis of a culturally accepted charisma was gradually eroded. By 1965 the phenomenon had become so widespread that Myerhoff and Larsen, viewing the medical profession as a whole, could predict that if the doctor is seen "in an increasingly prosaic light, he will lose his power to claim the patient's absolute confidence and in so doing will lose an essential ingredient of his success." Speaking of physicians generally, the authors go on to say that "we suspect that their occupational effectiveness will be impaired by their rapidly growing familiarity" (Barbara Myerhoff and William Larsen, "The Doctor as Culture Hero: The Routinization of Charisma," *Human Organization,* vol. 24, pp. 188–91, 1965).

By 1970 the average citizen was more likely to come across derogatory portrayals of physicians than praise-filled ones (see, e.g., *Our Ailing Medical System,* written by the editors of *Fortune* magazine, New York, Harper and Row, 1969; Daniel Schorr, *Don't Get Sick in America,* Nashville, Tenn., Aurora Publishers, 1970; Anselm Strauss, *Where Medicine Fails,* Brunswick, N.J., Transaction, Inc., 1970; Abraham Ribicoff, *The American Medical Machine,* New York, Harper and Row, 1973; Ivan Illich. *Medical Nemesis: The Expropriation of Health,* New York, Pantheon, 1976; and John Knowles et al., *Doing Better and Feeling Worse: Health in the United States,* New York, W. W. Norton, 1977).

Of all of medicine, psychiatry has been most widely and viciously criticized. As a political scientist and observer of the scene, Rogow commented that "in recent years the critics of psychiatrists and psychoanalysts have become almost as numerous as their patients, and even, in many instances, identical with them. *Books in Print* lists dozens of antipsychiatry works, not counting novels and plays, in which psychotherapists are depicted as sadists, lechers, psychopaths, or, at the very least, people as troubled as those who come to consult them (Arnold Rogow, "Shrink-Shrinking," *New York Times Book Review,* pp. 7, 33, April 23, 1978). For examples of the genre, one need only browse through any library (see, e.g., Dorothy Tenov, *Psychotherapy: The Hazardous Cure,* New York, Abelard-Schuman, 1975; Thomas Szasz, *Psychiatric Slavery,* New York, Free Press, 1977; Peter Schrag, *Mind Control,* New York, Pantheon, 1978; and Hugh Drummond, "You're Okay—They're Not," *Mother Jones,* pp. 19–22, April 1978). Particularly bruising was *The Death of Psychiatry,* leading many psychiatrists to ask "if psychiatry is dead, then what—and who—am I?" (E. Fuller Torrey, *The Death of Psychiatry,* New York,

Penguin Books, 1975). The impact on the profession has been predictable and is most vividly, though often superficially and misleadingly, portrayed for the general public in *Time* magazine's cover story, "Psychiatry's Depression" (*Time,* April 2, 1979).

The effect of the same events on the public included both the increase of demands on an individual and social policy levels. According to Thomas: "Nothing has changed so much in the health care system over the past twenty-five years as the public's perception of its own health. . . . There is a public preoccupation with disease that is assuming the dimensions of a national obsession. . . . Every mail brings word of the imminent perils posed by multiple sclerosis, kidney disease, cancer, heart disease, cystic fibrosis, asthma, muscular dystrophy, and the rest" (Lewis Thomas in Knowles, cited above, p. 43).

As the public's preoccupation has grown, the demand for convenient services likewise has grown: " 'Health delivery' became the catchword. At times it almost seemed as if the welcome wagon was supposed to roll up to the door and deliver health, wrapped in a neat package" (Aaron Wildavsky, in Knowles, cited above, p. 112).

Helms attributes rising health costs to the greater expense of labor, technology, and inflation generally, but also to "specific policies adopted by Congress to achieve alternative, and often quite popular, objectives." In this latter category, he includes various schemes to spread services more widely at lower direct cost to the consumer (e.g. Medicare, Medicaid) and "various tax subsidies that have distorted incentives in the medical care markets": deductions for medical expenses on standard income tax forms, incentives to unions and employees to bargain for nontaxable health insurance rather than taxable wages, etc. (Robert Helms, "The Health Care Problem: Is Regulation Our Only Hope?" *Proceedings of the New York Academy of Medicine,* Winter 1979–1980).

One doesn't have to read very far in the field of health-care economics to learn that there is an enormous range of figures available for practically every variable. My most useful sources have been the *Social Security Bulletin* and publications of the National Center for Health Statistics and the Center for Health Policy Studies. Practically the only thing that everyone agrees on is that the fiscal situation is terrible and getting worse. For example: "[The] massive infusion of federal funds, excess hospital capacity in some areas of the country, the inadequacy of incentives to use the less expensive service alternatives, the increased use and sophistication of resources, and a variety of other factors [have] contributed to virtually uncontrollable price increases in health services in recent years" (*The Federal Health Dollar 1969 to 1976,* Center for Health Policy Studies, 1977). Another typical comment is that "if money is a barrier to medicine, the system is discriminatory. If money is no barrier, the system gets over-crowded" (Wildavsky in Knowles, cited above, p. 111).

Typical examples of the public-opinion polls include the 1978 Lou Harris poll, wherein only 39 percent of those surveyed said they had "a great deal" of confidence in physicians, a drop of 34 points in twelve years, all of which seems to conflict with a University of Chicago survey, conducted the previous year, which revealed that "88 percent of respondents were satisfied with their last visit to a doctor" ("Doctors' Public Image Hits Twelve-Year Low," *Medical World News,* June 26, 1978).

16. TEAM CARE AND TEAM POLITICS

Information about the number and titles of health-industry occupations is available in a publication entitled *Health Resources Statistics* from the National Center for Health Statistics.

In the 95th Congress, Senator Inouye had three bills pending, designed to benefit both the nursing and social-work professions. None of them reached the floor for voting. The American Nurses Association is a fruitful source of information about the expanding role of nurses (see, e.g., the pamphlet entitled *Professional Development in Psychiatric and Mental Health Nursing,* Kansas City, Mo., American Nurses Association, 1975). That physicians other than psychiatrists are affected has been dramatically portrayed in a cover story of a widely circulated physicians' magazine (Reginald Rhein Jr., "Nurses: Colleagues or Competitors?" *Medical World News,* July 9, 1979), in which an apparently representative nurse practitioner is quoted as saying, "I can do anything a GP can do." Nurses, among others, are gaining strength in implementing their increasingly bold self-perceptions. The following is a representative example of the stance: "What the nurse can do in private practice is usually what the physician does in private practice. . . . Today, nurse leaders, primarily educators, strongly believe that the profession of nursing can unilaterally define its goals and can set its course of action to achieve these goals" (Ellen Davis and E. M. Pattison, "The Psychiatric Nurse's Role Identity," *American Journal of Nursing,* vol. 79, pp. 298–299, February 1979—see also, "Expanded Privileges for RN's, PA's Debated," *American Medical News,* pp. 1, 16–17, October 5, 1979).

Dorken and Whiting have published a thorough report of the expanding scope of psychologists in practice (Herbert Dorken and J. Frank Whiting, "Psychologists As Health Service Providers," *Professional Psychology,* vol. 5, pp. 309–319, August 1974; see also the three-part series concerning psychologists by Margaret McDonald, in *Psychiatric News,* October and November of 1977). The psychologists' territorial expansion has been accompanied by considerable internal turmoil, some of it at a conceptual level, but a lot having to do with battles over turf (John Walsh, "Professional Psychologists Seek to Change Roles," *Science,* vol. 203, pp. 338–340, January 26, 1979). In the process, psychologists themselves have often struggled with their own identity (Richard G. Weigel, "I Have Seen the Enemy and They Is Us—and Everyone Else," *The Counseling Psychologist,* vol. 7, pp. 50–53, 1977) and with much of the same criticism that is directed at psychiatry (Martin Gross, *The Psychological Society,* New York, Random House, 1978).

Lubove has written a fascinating account of the development of social work as a career, replete with sociologic jargon, but providing penetrating insight into the history of professionalized benevolence (Roy Lubove, *The Professional Altruist—The Emergence of Social Work as a Career, 1880-1930,* Cambridge, Mass., Harvard University Press, 1965). The social-work literature is filled with analyses of the profession's problems. One typical example begins by saying that "difficult times are evoking in social workers an agonizing elusive quest for a professional identity" (Richard Grinnell, Jr., and Nancy Kyte, "The Future of Clincial Practice: A Study," *Clinical Social Work Journal,* vol. 5, pp. 132–138, Summer 1977).

For a thorough review of the history and present status of the doctorate of mental health program, see Margaret McDonald's three-part series in *Psychiatric News,* March and April 1978. All information concerning marriage and family counselors, the American Association of Sex Educators, Counselors, and Therapists, psychiatric technicians, music therapists, art therapists, and dance therapists has been drawn from the brochures of their respective professional organizations. Pattison and Elpers examine the multiplicity of professions from a national manpower perspective (Mansell Pattison and John Elpers, "A Developmental View of Mental Health Manpower Trends," *Hospital and Community Psychiatry*, vol. 23, pp. 325–328, November 1972) and McPheeters puts the two-year-college-trained workers into historical perspective (Harold McPheeters, "The Middle Level Mental Health Worker: His Training," *Hospital and Community Psychiatry*, vol. 23, pp. 334–335, November 1972). The relationship between psychiatrists and co-workers has been the subject of an unending stream of articles (see, e.g., Elliott Heiman, "The Future Relationship of Psychiatrists with Other Mental Health Professionals," *Psychiatric Opinion*, vol. 15, pp. 25–30, October 1978; and William C. House, et al., "Role Definitions Among Mental Health Professionals," *Comprehensive Psychiatry*, vol. 19, pp. 469–476, September/October 1978).

Territorial struggles in medicine generally—as opposed to the mental-health arena specifically—have been percolating to public attention more quietly, but are certainly no less fascinating. Rayack gave an excellent early account, though approaching the topic in another context (see, e.g., Ch. 4, "The Shortage of Physicians," and Ch. 6, "Medical Imperialism: Conflict Among the Health Professions," in Elton Rayack, *Professional Power and American Medicine: The Economics of the American Medical Association*, Cleveland, Ohio, World Publishing Co. 1967). Ryan observed the obvious trend, and used an editorial format for a worried call to action (Allan Ryan, "Are Physicians Giving Away Their Profession?" *Postgraduate Medicine*, vol. 63, pp. 17–18, March 1978).

See also Wilensky's article for a scholarly overview of the entire subject as it relates to such nonmedical professionals as professors, lawyers, and engineers (Harold Wilensky, "The Professionalization of Everyone?" *American Journal of Sociology*, vol. 70, pp. 137–158, September 1964).

Hans Eysenck was an early critic of the evidence used to document psychotherapy's effectiveness (H. J. Eysenck, "The Effects of Psychotherapy: An Evaluation," *Journal of Consulting Psychology*, vol. 16, pp. 319–24, 1952). His point then, and more recently too, was that there has never been a single adequate experimental study that supported the unique curative effects of psychotherapy (see also Allen Bergin, "Some Implications of Psychotherapy Research for Therapeutic Practice," *Journal of Abnormal Psychology,* vol. 71, pp. 235–46, 1966; David Malan, "The Outcome Problem in Psychotherapy Research—A Historical Review," *Archives of General Psychiatry,* vol. 29, pp. 719–729, December 1973; and Lester Luborsky et al., "Comparative Studies of Psychotherapies: Is It True That 'Everyone Has Won and All Must Have Prizes'?" *Archives of General Psychiatry,* vol. 32, pp. 995–1008, August 1975). One study which I found particularly depressing was a thirty-year follow-up of delinquency-prone boys, comparing those who underwent a five-year-long treatment program with controls. The results indicate that "the program had negative side effects as measured by criminal behavior, death, disease, occupational status, and job satisfaction." The author concludes that "the program seems not only to have failed to prevent its clients from committing crimes . . . but also to have produced negative side effects" (Joan McCord, "A 30-Year Followup of Treatment Effects," *American Psychologist,* pp. 284–289, March 1978). She is quoted elsewhere as saying that her results "indicate that some of the most widely held beliefs about therapy may be untenable."

There was enormous interest in disease classification in psychiatry near the turn of the century, largely deriving from the conviction that better classification would lead to better understanding and better remedies. Classification for the sake of defining professional boundaries and determining fees—Gibson uses the term *acute reimbursable reaction*—is a more recent phenomenon (Robert Gibson, "Survival of the Most Reimbursable," *NAPPH Journal,* vol. 9, pp. 33–35). An account of disagreements between psychiatrists and psychologists over the issue is available from a variety of sources (see, e.g., *Psychiatric News,* pp. 1, 14–15, December 2, 1977). Some of the more colorful discussions occur around the exclusion of homosexuality from the current nomenclature (Charles Socarides, "The Sexual Deviations and the Diagnostic Manual," *American Journal of Psychotherapy,* vol. 32, pp. 414–426, July 1978) and the inclusion of some patterns of tobacco usage ("Jaffe Defends Disorder Label for Habitual Smokers," *Psychiatric News,* pp. 35, 39a, October 6, 1978).

The dramatic growth of the consumer movement is so well known that it requires no documentation here. Haug and Sussman review the trends and their implications for the professional and conclude on an optimistic note: "What the client demands—the professional as a limited consultant—may be less a curse than a blessing in disguise. It could enable the professional to give up the 'whole man' approach to service and treatment, and enable him to revert to a more specialized expert role" (Marie Haug and Marvin Sussman, "Professional Autonomy and the Revolt of the Client," *Social Problems,* vol. 17, pp. 153–161, Fall 1969; see also Leo Reeder, "The Patient-Client As a Consumer: Some Observations on the Changing Professional-Client Relationship," *Journal of Health and Social Behavior,* vol. 13, pp. 406–12, 1972). Stacey worries that applying the word *consumer* to patients at once undervalues and oversimplifies: "not only is the health service [in Britain] much more than economic enterprise, insofar as one does think of the health service as an industry, a patient can be said to be a producer as much as a consumer of that elusive and abstract good: health" (Margaret Stacey, "The Health Service Consumer: A Sociological Misconception," *Sociological Review,* pp. 194–200, 1976).

I first came across the term *burn-out* in relation to health professionals in a 1970 article by Burton (Arthur Burton, "The Adoration of the Patient and Its Disillusionment," *American Journal of Psychoanalysis,* vol. 29, pp. 194–204, 1970). Freudenberger contributed another early article (Herbert Freudenberger, "The Staff Burn-Out Syndrome in Alternative Institutions," *Psychotherapy: Theory, Research, and Practice,* vol. 12, pp. 73–82, Spring 1975). One chilling report suggests that clinical experience and a few gray hairs, rather than giving clinicians perspective and greater resistance to burn-out, tends to add cynicism and despair. The report says: "The longer staff had worked in the mental health field, the less they liked working with patients, the less accessible they felt with them, the more custodial rather than humanistic were their attitudes toward mental illness. They stopped looking for self-fulfillment in work, good days became infrequent, and the only good things about their work were the job conditions" (Ayala Pines and Christina Maslach, "Characteristics of Staff Burn-Out in Mental Health Settings," *Hospital and Community Psychiatry,* vol. 29, pp. 233–237, April 1978). The literature on the subject is expanding rapidly (see, e.g., Charles Larson, et al., "Therapist Burn-Out: Perspectives on a Critical Issue," *Social Casework,* pp. 563–565, November 1978; and Frank Devine, "A Hospital Psychologist Responds to an Analysis of Staff Burn-Out, *Hospital and Community Psychiatry,* vol. 29, p. 683, October 1978).

17. A PROGNOSIS FOR THE DOCTOR-PATIENT RELATIONSHIP

My own predictions for medicine's future may seem bleak to some, but I am by no means alone in my forecast. Whatever the virtues of the National Health Service in Britain—and I will acknowledge many—there can be no doubt about some of the deleterious effects of bureaucratization: "The living power of medicine, resident as it has always been, and must be, in the personnel of the profession, has passed out of its hands to be lost in the dead machinery of the bureau. Medicine has become what we pledged ourselves it never should become—a branch of the civil service. We are no longer experts. We sit and sign forms" (Lord Horder in E. S. Turner, *Call the Doctor*, p. 307, New York, St. Martin's Press, 1959). Kass, a research professor in bioethics, maintains that "once the definition of health care and the standards of medical practice are made by outsiders—and the national health insurance schemes all tend in this direction—the physician becomes a mere technician" (Leon Kass, "Regarding the End of Medicine and the Pursuit of Health," *The Public Interest*, vol. 40, pp. 11–43, Summer 1975). Fuchs portrays the future with an analogy: "That some physicians will continue to practice in traditional ways there can be no doubt. But this should be given no more weight than the fact that some custom tailors and dressmakers survive in an economy in which most people buy their clothing ready made" (Victor Fuchs, "Can the Traditional Practice of Medicine Survive?" *Archives of Internal Medicine*, vol. 125, pp. 154–176, January 1970). Maxmen states his sweeping predictions as an advocate: "We are entering into a new medical era—an era I believe will culminate in the total obsolescence of the physician. . . . In the future all of the functions currently performed by physicians can be accomplished by a partnership of paraprofessionals and computers." Although he looks forward to such eventualities, he says that all will not be bliss: "Despite its numerous advantages, a Post-Physician Era will not become a medical utopia. Illness, Kafkaesque bureaucracies, inadequate continuity of care, impersonal practitioners, and violations of confidentiality may continue to disturb patients. Improper priorities, fiscal problems, widespread resistance to organizational restructuring, consumer demands, and political pressures may continue to plague administrators. Malpractice suits, governmental interventions, and legal restrictions may continue to harass health care personnel. Although these problems will persist, they are not unmanageable" (Jerrold Maxmen, *The Post-Physician Era: Medicine in the 21st Century,* pp. 15–16, 93, New York, John Wiley and Sons, 1976).

Chapman, a professor of medicine and former president of the American Heart Association, says, "My own state of mind in these discouraging times is probably on the gloomy side of dead center.... All of us in the health professions are on the spot together; and together we must, no matter how trying things get, keep the focus on excellence in education and in the services we deliver. Otherwise the ultimate prospect is worse than gloomy" (Carlton Chapman, "Politics and the Health Professions—With Special Reference to Medical Education," *The Pharos,* vol. 32, pp. 70–74, July 1969).

For a discouraging view of the morale of the largest nonphysician professional group involved in health care, read Kramer's account of the conflict between bureaucratic requirements and professional ideals in nursing (Marlene Kramer, *Reality Shock: Why Nurses Leave Nursing,* New York, C. V. Mosby, 1974). The expanding "burn-out" literature also provides some valuable insights to issues of morale in the human services professions (see *Child Care Quarterly,* vol. 4, pp. 90–99, Summer 1977, which includes the following articles: Herbert Freudenberger, "Burnout—Occupational Hazard of the Childcare Worker"; Martha Mattingly, "Sources of Stress and Burn-out in Professional Childcare Work," pp. 127–137; and Christina Maslach and Ayala Pines, "The Burnout Syndrome in the Daycare Setting" pp. 100–113).

Maslach and Pines say that "the source of the problem is not the individual but the structure and the environment of the helping professions themselves.... The helping professions are asked to be warm and caring, on the one hand, and objective, on the other. If they fail to meet these high expectations and treat their patients or clients in ways that are considered indifferent, rude, or even dehumanizing, people are quick to criticize them and complain about the individuals who staff society's service institutions" (Chapter entitled "Burn-Out: The Loss of Human Caring," in Ayala Pines and Christina Maslach, *Experiencing Social Psychology,* p. 246, New York: Knopf, 1979).

18. NOTES TO WOULD-BE HEALERS

One of the fascinating developments in recent years, especially in the past decade, is the growing literature of physician introspection, especially in psychiatry. McCarley reports on psychiatrists who use a group format for this purpose (Tracey McCarley, "The Psychotherapist's Search for Self-Renewal," *American Journal of Psychiatry,* vol. 132. pp. 221–224, March 1975). Others have contributed penetrating analyses (see, e.g., Roy Menninger, "Psychiatrists' Identity: Quo Vadis?" *Bulletin of the Menninger Clinic,* vol. 42, pp. 138–43, 1968; Judd Marmor, "The Psychoanalyst As a Person," *The American Journal of Psychoanalysis,* vol. 37, pp. 275–84, 1977; and James Spensley and K. H. Blacker, "Feelings of the Psychotherapist," *American Journal of Orthopsychiatry,* vol. 46, pp. 542–545, July 1976).

Coles has contributed several useful articles, concluding in an early one: "I would hope that we would dare to accept ourselves fully and offer ourselves freely to a quizzical and apprehensive time and to uneasy and restless people" (Robert Coles, "A Young Psychiatrist Looks at His Profession," in Charles Rolo, ed., *Psychiatry in American Life,* pp. 102–113, Boston, Mass., Little, Brown, 1963; see also Coles, "The End of the Affair," *Katallagate—Journal of the Committee of Southern Churchmen,* pp. 46–58, Fall/Winter 1972).

A number of highly provocative pieces concentrate on the risks inherent in being a clinician (see, e.g., Richard Chessick, "The Sad Soul of the Psychiatrist," *Bulletin of the Menninger Clinic,* vol. 42, pp. 1–9, January 1978; John Spiegel, "Psychiatry—A High-Risk Profession," *American Journal of Psychiatry,* vol. 132, pp. 693–697, July 1975; and Ch. 7, "The Vocational Hazards of Psychoanalysis," in Allen Wheelis, *A Quest for Identity,* New York, W. W. Norton, 1958). Lederer counsels a younger colleague to "be sure you add to that pipe, behind which you now hide, some warm slippers, and a warm hearth, and the unhurried warmth of loving arms. You, who will have to mother so many, marry for heaven sakes a woman who, if needed, won't shrink from mothering you; listen to the cry of *your own* children; cultivate *your own* garden; enjoy and suffer *your own* attachments and involvements: lest you lose your footing, and get swept away—lest you become a premature actuarial statistic . . . ." (Wolfgang Lederer, "Stalking the Demons: A Psychiatrist Reflects on His Resident," *The Progressive,* September 1967). Rosen too suggests balancing the demands of professional life with avocational pursuits (David Rosen, "The Pursuit of One's Own Healing," *American Journal of Psychoanalysis,* vol. 37, pp. 37–41, 1977). Yager recommends "pragmatic skepticism" to psychiatrists in training (Joel Yager, "A Survival Guide for Psychiatric Residents," *Archives of General Psychiatry,* vol. 30, pp. 494–499, April 1974).

The literature concerning nonpsychiatric physicians is no less voluminous, though it tends to focus more on external hazards than internal psychodynamics (see, e.g., the cover story by Malcolm Manber, "Being A Doctor May Be Hazardous to Your Health," *Medical World News,* August 20, 1979). In 1977 the American Academy of Family Practice began presenting a series of workshops in various parts of the country entitled "Learning to Cope with Practice Pressures: The Needs of Physicians, Their Families, and Their Patients." Various other organizations and publications have similarly responded to what is perceived as a growing need.

Mawardi (cited in the Notes, Chapter 12) observes that "many of the new sources of stress that are being heard today [among the physicians studied] relate to a breakdown in the traditional physician-patient relationship" (see also Samual Guze, "Can the Practice of Medicine Be Fun for a Lifetime?" *JAMA,* Vol. 241, pp. 2021–2023, May 11, 1979).

That physicians are not alone in having lost the secure feeling of respect in the eyes of the public has been widely documented. Kirsch maintains that " . . . expertise is the fallen idol of the sixties" (Jonathan Kirsch, "Pity the Poor Expert," *New West Magazine,* p. 100, July 3, 1978).

Margaret Mead commented along the same lines: "There is a questioning all over the world, by colonialized peoples, by minorities, by women, of an order of life in which others—teachers, administrators, social workers, members of other classes and races, and of the other sex—care for them, no matter how well intentioned that care might be" *(New York Times,* p. 51, January 12, 1974).

Barzun says that "not only physicians—but lawyers, scientists, and academics—are facing the disillusionment of a fickle public. . . . Without some . . . heroic effort, we professionals shall all go down— appropriately—as non-heroes together" (Jacques Barzun, "The Medical Profession Under Fire," *Impact/American Medical News,* pp. 1–2, May 25, 1979).

INDEX